The Art of Goat Milk Soap Making

MORGAN DESPIEGELAERE

ISBN 978-1-964165-80-6

Dedication

To my husband, thank you for everything you do that allows me to do the things that I love.

To my son, for always thinking my slightly crazy ideas are the best and for being my right-hand man.

To my daughter, for always cheering me on and being mommy's number one fan.

Love you forever.

Contents

Author's Note

My passion for goat milk soap-making began shortly after I had my first child. As I adjusted to motherhood, I found myself searching for a creative outlet that could be directly linked to my livestock– something that allowed me to nurture my artistic side while also benefiting my family. That's when I discovered the magic of goat milk soap. It quickly became more than just a hobby; it became a way to express creativity, connect with nature, and provide natural, nourishing skincare.

In crafting my recipes, I carefully selected oils and ingredients that worked best for me, my family's skin, and what was available to me. I encourage you to do the same. Every batch of soap can be tailored to your needs and preferences, making it a truly personal experience.

I hope this book serves as a helpful guide to get you started on your own goat milk soap-making journey and that it brings you the same sense of joy, creativity, and fulfillment that it has brought me. Whether you are making soap for personal use, gifts, or to start your own business, I believe this craft has something special to offer everyone.

Enjoy the process, embrace the creativity, and most of all, have fun with it!

Chapter One:
Introduction to Soap Making
—The Beauty of Making Your Own Soap

Soap making is an ancient craft, an art form that has evolved through centuries but remains as essential and beloved as ever. Though we often take soap for granted today, relegating it to a mere household necessity, its origins tell a much richer story—one that intertwines with the evolution of societies and their resources. From the rudimentary soap-like substances discovered in ancient Babylon to the highly refined, perfumed soaps of medieval Europe, this humble product has always served an essential purpose: cleanliness, care, and healing.

The first records of soap-making date back over 5,000 years, to the Mesopotamians, who used a combination of water, alkali, and cassia oil. Similarly, the ancient Egyptians had their own formulas for soap, using animal fats mixed with alkaline salts to wash their bodies and treat skin diseases. Soap wasn't just a luxury item for royalty but was also used by everyday people to maintain hygiene. In places like Rome, soap became a staple of their famed public bathhouses, although it was initially viewed with some skepticism for its medicinal properties.

As the world entered the Industrial Revolution, soap making moved from a domestic craft into large-scale production. The proliferation of soap factories in the 19th century made soap more accessible to the masses, but this shift also led to a significant change in the ingredients used. Commercial soap makers, in pursuit of lower costs and longer shelf life, began to replace the natural oils and fats once used with synthetic ingredients and harsh chemicals. This change created a divide between traditional, handmade soap and the mass-produced alternatives we see today.

While commercial soaps are undeniably convenient, many contain sulfates, parabens, artificial dyes, and synthetic fragrances—all of which can strip the skin of its natural moisture and cause irritation, especially for those with sensitive skin. In response, the art of handmade soap has been resurrected in recent years by homesteaders, artisans, and those who desire a more natural approach to skincare. In particular, goat milk soap has emerged as a standout choice, offering a luxurious and deeply nourishing option for the skin.

Goat Milk Soap and the Sustainable Homestead

For the homesteader, goat milk is a resource of both sustenance and opportunity. Many homesteads keep goats for their milk, enjoying the fresh, creamy taste and the health benefits that come with it. But goat milk is not just for drinking or making cheese; it can also be used to create skin-nourishing soap. By incorporating goat milk into soap recipes, homesteaders can take advantage of every drop of milk produced on their farm, ensuring that nothing goes to waste.

One of the most beautiful aspects of homesteading is the ability to transform raw materials into useful products. Goat milk, combined with natural oils and essential oils, can be turned into a soap that's not only beneficial for the skin but also aligns with a sustainable way of life. Goat milk soap allows homesteaders to create something valuable from what they already have on hand—a testament to the ingenuity and resourcefulness that defines homestead living.

Making your own soap, especially from the milk of your goats, is more than just a creative project; it's a step toward self-sufficiency. Each bar of soap represents a cycle of sustainability. The goats are fed and cared for on the farm, their milk is harvested, and that milk is then used to make soap, providing a natural, chemical-free alternative to store-bought cleaners. There's a deep sense of fulfillment in knowing that what you create with your hands can replace commercial products that are often loaded with synthetic additives and chemicals.

More than just a skincare product, goat milk soap fits perfectly within the broader philosophy of homesteading—living lightly on the land, reducing waste, and using natural resources efficiently. Each bar becomes a small but significant contribution to a lifestyle centered around sustainability and self-reliance. When you craft soap from your own goat's milk, you aren't just making soap; you're making a statement about the kind of life you want to live.

The Appeal of Handmade Soap over Commercial Products

In today's fast-paced, convenience-driven world, making your own soap might seem unnecessary at first glance. With every drugstore aisle lined with endless options for skincare products, why would anyone bother with the time and effort involved in creating soap from scratch? The answer lies in the growing awareness of the potential dangers lurking in commercial products.

Most commercial soaps are not true soaps but are classified as detergents. They are made from synthetic ingredients designed to create lather quickly, but these ingredients can be harsh and dry to the skin. Common ingredients like sodium lauryl sulfate (SLS) and artificial fragrances can cause irritation, disrupt the skin's natural pH balance, and contribute to skin conditions such as eczema and dermatitis. Moreover, many commercial soaps contain preservatives and chemicals that allow them to sit on store shelves for months or even years.

Handmade soap, by contrast, is made using natural ingredients that nourish the skin. Goat milk, in particular, is rich in lactic acid, which acts as a gentle exfoliant, helping to remove dead skin cells and promote the growth of new ones. It also contains fatty acids that help to hydrate and repair the skin, making it an excellent choice for those with dry or sensitive skin. Combined with natural oils like olive oil, coconut oil, and shea butter, goat milk soap offers a luxurious and moisturizing experience that commercial soaps simply cannot match.

Beyond the ingredients, there's something deeply satisfying about the process of making soap by hand. It's a creative outlet that allows you to control every aspect of what goes into the product. You can choose the oils, scents, and additives that best suit your skin's needs, and you can experiment with different textures, colors, and shapes. Every batch of handmade soap is unique, a reflection of the maker's creativity and care.

Handmade soap also carries a personal touch that commercial products lack. When you make your own soap, you're not just crafting a product; you're creating something that tells a story. Each bar represents the time, effort, and love that went into its creation. For many people, using handmade soap is a way to reconnect with a simpler, more mindful way of living—one that values quality, craftsmanship, and the natural world.

My Journey: From Family Sensitivities to Soap Maker

What started out as getting goats to milk to feed my son, who had a sensitive tummy, turned into producing more goat milk than we could consume. The idea of turning that surplus milk into soap seemed like the perfect solution. I started experimenting with basic recipes, using simple ingredients like olive oil and coconut oil. The results were astonishing. Not only was the soap incredibly moisturizing, but it also soothed the sensitive skin in a way that no commercial product had ever done. My entire family, being sensitive to store-bought soaps with way too much fake scent and synthetic ingredients, has benefited immensely.

From there, my soap-making hobby grew. I started sharing my handmade goat milk soap with friends and family, who quickly became enthusiastic fans. They loved the gentle, creamy lather and the way the soap left their skin feeling soft and nourished. Word spread, and soon, I found myself making larger batches to meet the growing demand. It wasn't long before I began selling my soap at local farmers' markets and craft fairs, turning what had started as a personal project into a small business.

Goat Milk Soap as a Business Opportunity

Starting a goat milk soap business has been an incredibly rewarding experience. Not only did it allow me to put my homestead resources to good use, but it also opened the door to new opportunities for creativity and growth. I began experimenting with different recipes, incorporating herbs and botanicals from my garden, such as lavender, chamomile, and calendula, to create soaps with added therapeutic benefits. The more I learned about soap making, the more I realized just how versatile and customizable it could be.

Running a small business out of my homestead came with its own set of challenges, but it also provided me with a sense of fulfillment that I hadn't anticipated. Every bar of soap I sold was a testament to the hard work and care that went into its creation. I loved hearing from customers who told me how much they enjoyed using the soap or how it had helped alleviate their skin issues. Knowing that I was providing people with a natural, handmade alternative to commercial products made the effort worthwhile.

As my business grew, so did my passion for soap making. I began to dive deeper into the craft, learning about the science behind saponification, experimenting with different ingredients, and perfecting my techniques. I also explored the legalities of selling handmade soap, particularly in Canada, where regulations require soap makers to adhere to specific guidelines for labeling and ingredient disclosure. Understanding these requirements became an essential part of running my business and ensuring that my products met all the necessary safety standards.

The Reward of Creating Practical Beauty

One of the most rewarding aspects of making goat milk soap is the ability to create something both beautiful and practical. Soap is a necessity, something that everyone uses daily, but when you make it yourself, it becomes more than just a functional item. Handmade goat milk soap is a work of art, a reflection of the care, creativity, and passion that went into its creation.

As homesteaders, we take pride in being able to provide for ourselves and our families using the resources from our land. Goat milk soap is a perfect example of this ethos—taking something as simple as milk and turning it into a luxurious, nourishing product that enhances our well-being. It's a reminder of the beauty that can be found in everyday life and the satisfaction that comes from creating something with your own hands.

Chapter Two:
Benefits of Goat Milk Soap

Not all soaps are created equal. While commercial soaps are abundant and convenient, they often leave your skin feeling tight, dry, or even irritated. Goat milk soap stands out as a nourishing, natural alternative with a range of benefits that support healthy skin. Rich in vitamins, minerals, and fatty acids, it offers a gentle, moisturizing cleanse while steering clear of the harsh chemicals often found in store-bought varieties. For those seeking skincare products that genuinely improve the skin's condition and provide holistic well-being, goat milk soap proves to be a powerful ally.

Nutrient-Rich Composition: Vitamins and Fatty Acids

Goat milk contains an impressive list of nutrients that directly benefit the skin. Its natural composition includes essential vitamins such as A, B1, B6, B12, C, D, and E, along with fatty acids, proteins, and minerals like zinc, selenium, and calcium. Vitamin A, known for its role in cell turnover, helps repair damaged skin and supports the maintenance of a youthful appearance. When used consistently, goat milk soap can contribute to smoother, healthier-looking skin by encouraging natural regeneration.

The fatty acids in goat milk are particularly significant. Fats such as capric, caprylic, and caproic acid help maintain the skin's moisture barrier, preventing water loss and improving elasticity. Many commercial soaps contain detergents that strip the skin of its natural oils, leaving it vulnerable to dryness. In contrast, the fats in goat milk soap work to replenish and lock in moisture, making it ideal for people with dry, sensitive, or mature skin.

Another key nutrient in goat milk is lactic acid. As a gentle alpha hydroxy acid (AHA), lactic acid naturally exfoliates the skin by dissolving dead skin cells, promoting cell renewal, and enhancing skin texture. Over time, regular use of goat milk soap can reduce the appearance of fine lines and uneven skin tone without the harshness associated with chemical exfoliants.

Alleviating Skin Issues: Eczema, Psoriasis, and Dry Skin

Goat milk soap is often recommended for individuals suffering from common skin conditions, such as eczema, psoriasis, and chronic dryness. Eczema, characterized by inflamed, itchy patches of skin, often worsens when exposed to soaps containing artificial fragrances and sulfates. Goat milk soap, with its natural anti-inflammatory properties, can help soothe irritation and reduce redness.

Psoriasis, a condition that causes the skin to develop thick, scaly patches, also responds well to the moisturizing effects of goat milk. While it is not a cure for psoriasis, the soap's ability to maintain the skin's moisture barrier can help alleviate symptoms and prevent flare-ups triggered by dryness. Many users report that the soap leaves their skin feeling calm and hydrated, making it an effective part of a gentle skincare routine.

Dry skin is a widespread issue, especially in colder climates or during winter months when humidity levels drop. Commercial soaps can exacerbate the problem by stripping away the skin's natural oils, leaving it dehydrated. Goat milk soap offers a gentler option, replenishing moisture while cleansing the skin without irritation. Its rich, creamy lather leaves the skin feeling soft and nourished, not tight or dry.

A Comparison with Commercial Soaps

A common complaint among users of commercial soap is the dryness and irritation that can result from regular use. Many mass-produced soaps rely on synthetic surfactants such as sodium lauryl sulfate (SLS) to create lather. While these agents produce the bubbles, many people associate with cleanliness, they are also known to strip the skin of its natural oils, leaving it exposed to environmental stressors.

In contrast, goat milk soap produces a luxurious, creamy lather without the need for synthetic surfactants. Its natural fats and proteins bind with impurities on the skin, gently lifting dirt and oils without disrupting the skin's protective barrier. This makes it particularly suitable for those with delicate or reactive skin who cannot tolerate the ingredients commonly found in conventional products.

Another advantage of goat milk soap is its lack of artificial fragrances and colorants. Many commercial soaps contain synthetic fragrances that can irritate the skin and cause allergic reactions. Goat milk soap, when scented with natural essential oils, offers a subtle fragrance without the risks associated with artificial chemicals. Users can also opt for unscented varieties, making it an excellent choice for individuals with allergies or hypersensitive skin.

Free from Harmful Chemicals and Additives

One of the greatest appeals of goat milk soap is its simple, natural ingredient list. With only a handful of core ingredients–such as goat milk, olive oil, coconut oil, and essential oils–this soap avoids the harmful additives often found in commercial products. Many store-bought soaps contain parabens, phthalates, and other preservatives linked to health concerns, including hormonal disruption and skin irritation.

Choosing goat milk soap means embracing a cleaner alternative that prioritizes skin health and well-being. By steering clear of synthetic chemicals, users can reduce their exposure to potential toxins and enjoy a more natural skincare routine. This makes goat milk soap especially beneficial for families, children, and individuals with chronic skin conditions who need a gentle, non-toxic product.

Testimonials and Real-Life Experiences

Over the years, countless individuals have experienced the transformative effects of switching to goat milk soap. For some, the change has been life-altering. A mother recalls her frustration with finding a suitable soap for her daughter, who struggled with eczema from infancy. "We tried everything," she explains, "but most soaps made her skin worse. Then, a friend recommended goat milk soap, and within a few weeks, her skin was noticeably calmer. It became a game-changer for us."

Others have shared similar success stories. A farmer in northern Canada discovered goat milk soap after battling dry, cracked hands for years. "Working outdoors in harsh winters takes a toll on your skin," he says. "But since I started using goat milk soap, my hands are no longer sore or cracked. I even keep a bar in the barn now."

These testimonials highlight the versatility of goat milk soap and its ability to improve various skin issues. From young children with sensitive skin to adults managing chronic dryness, the soap provides a gentle, reliable solution. Many users also note that the switch to handmade soap has inspired them to adopt other natural skincare practices, enhancing their overall well-being.

Holistic Benefits: Mental Relaxation and Mindful Living

Beyond its physical benefits, using goat milk soap offers a form of mental relaxation. There is something inherently calming about knowing that the products you use on your skin are crafted with care and free from harmful chemicals. Each bar of goat milk soap carries a subtle reminder that skin care can be simple, pure, and effective.

The act of washing with handmade soap becomes a small but meaningful ritual that encourages mindfulness and self-care. The silky lather, soft texture, and natural scents promote a sense of relaxation, turning an ordinary routine into a moment of tranquility. In a world where we are often overwhelmed by stress and fast-paced living, these small moments of self-care can make a significant difference to mental health.

Many soap makers and customers alike describe the experience of using goat milk soap as grounding. The connection to natural ingredients, combined with the simplicity of the product, reinforces a sense of harmony with nature. This is particularly true for those who make the soap themselves, as they experience the joy of creating something beautiful and practical from raw materials.

A Gentle and Nourishing Choice

Aside from offering a cleanse, goat milk soap also provides nourishment, comfort, and care for the skin. Its nutrient-rich formula helps alleviate common skin conditions, while its gentle cleansing action makes it suitable for even the most sensitive skin types. Free from synthetic chemicals, the soap provides a natural alternative to commercial products, promoting healthier skin and mindful living.

The testimonials from satisfied users demonstrate the profound impact this simple product can have on daily life. Whether you're managing eczema, combating dryness, or simply seeking a natural skincare option, goat milk soap offers a solution that works. In choosing goat milk soap, you are not only caring for your skin but also embracing a lifestyle that values simplicity, sustainability, and well-being.

As we continue exploring the many facets of goat milk soap in this book, you'll discover how easy it is to incorporate this nourishing product into your routine and perhaps even inspire others to make the switch. After all, the journey toward healthier skin begins with a single bar.

Chapter Three:
Equipment Needed

Making goat milk soap at home is both an art and a science, requiring precision, attention to detail, and the right tools. While the ingredients you choose are critical to producing high-quality soap, the equipment you use plays an equally important role in ensuring safety and success. In this chapter, we'll explore the essential equipment needed for soap making, discuss the function of each tool, and provide tips for sourcing affordable supplies. Whether you're a beginner or an experienced soap maker, understanding the importance of each item will help you create a safe, efficient, and enjoyable soap-making process.

Core Equipment: The Basics

When embarking on the soap-making journey, there are a few key pieces of equipment you'll need. These tools not only make the process more manageable but also ensure that your measurements and temperatures are accurate, leading to a better final product. Below is a list of essential equipment and why each item is necessary:

1. Molds

Soap molds are an absolute must in the soap-making process, as they give your bars their shape and structure. Molds come in various materials, such as silicone, wood, and plastic, each offering distinct advantages. Silicone molds are flexible and non-stick, making them easy to use and clean. Wooden molds, on the other hand, provide excellent insulation during the curing process, which can affect the texture of the soap. Plastic molds, while less popular, can be useful for beginners due to their affordability and wide variety of shapes.

The type of mold you choose will also influence the final appearance of your soap. Simple rectangular molds are perfect for standard bars, while more intricate molds can create decorative shapes, adding a creative touch to your products. For a homesteader looking to produce practical yet appealing soap, investing in good quality molds is highly recommended. Over time, you can even create your own custom molds, adding a unique signature to your soap-making endeavors.

2. Digital Scale

Accuracy is paramount when it comes to soap making, and a reliable digital scale is essential for measuring ingredients. Unlike cooking or baking, soap-making requires precise measurements–

especially when working with lye, which must be accurately balanced with fats and oils. Too little or too much of any ingredient can affect the texture, hardness, and lather of the soap. A digital scale ensures that you are working with exact amounts, which will help produce consistent results.

A kitchen scale that measures in grams and ounces is ideal, as you'll often need to work with small amounts of ingredients. Avoid using a mechanical or manual scale, as they tend to be less precise. Remember, even a minor discrepancy in measurement can change the outcome of your batch, so invest in a good-quality digital scale to avoid unnecessary mishaps.

3. Thermometer

In soap making, temperature control is critical to ensuring the lye and oils combine smoothly. Using a thermometer allows you to monitor the temperature of your lye solution and oils before mixing them together. The temperature of both liquids should be within a specific range–typically between 90°F and 110°F (32°C to 43°C)–to avoid problems like separation or uneven texture in your final product.

An infrared thermometer is often the most convenient option, as it allows you to check temperatures quickly without immersing the device in the liquid. However, a simple candy or meat thermometer can also suffice as long as it provides accurate readings. Whichever option you choose, keep it designated for soap-making to prevent cross-contamination with food items.

4. Stick Blender (Immersion Blender)

While you can stir your soap mixture by hand, using a stick blender speeds up the process considerably. Once your lye solution and oils are mixed, the blend must reach "trace"–a stage where the mixture thickens and leaves visible lines on the surface when drizzled. Achieving trace by hand can take up to an hour or more, depending on the recipe, but a stick blender reduces this time to just a few minutes.

Stick blenders are inexpensive and easy to use, making them a staple in any soap maker's toolkit. Be sure to use a blender with a stainless-steel shaft, as plastic models may not withstand the caustic properties of lye. As with the thermometer, designate this tool solely for soap-making to avoid contamination.

Safety Equipment: Protecting Yourself

Handling lye (sodium hydroxide) is an essential but potentially dangerous part of soap making. Lye is a caustic substance that can cause chemical burns or injury if it comes into contact with your skin, eyes, or lungs. Therefore, it's crucial to have proper safety equipment on hand to protect yourself during the process. Below are the safety tools you should never skip:

1. Gloves

Nitrile or rubber gloves are a must when working with lye and soap batter. They protect your skin from the corrosive effects of lye, which can cause severe burns if it comes into contact with bare skin. Always wear gloves during the soap-making process, from mixing the lye to pouring the soap into molds. Make sure your gloves fit snugly but comfortably, allowing you to handle equipment and ingredients with precision.

2. Goggles

Protecting your eyes is equally important when working with lye, as even a small splash can cause serious damage. Safety goggles should be worn at all times when handling lye or mixing the soap batter. Choose goggles that provide full coverage, preventing lye or soap from splashing into your eyes. Some soap makers opt for face shields for additional protection, especially when working with larger batches.

3. Long-Sleeved Shirt and Apron

Wearing a long-sleeved shirt and an apron adds an extra layer of protection for your skin and clothing. This is particularly important during the mixing phase when lye is most dangerous. A long-sleeved shirt minimizes the risk of accidental splashes on your arms, while an apron protects your clothing from lye and soap batter.

4. Proper Ventilation

Lye emits fumes when mixed with water, which can irritate your respiratory system. Always mix lye in a well-ventilated area, preferably near an open window or outdoors. If you are particularly sensitive to fumes, consider wearing a mask to minimize exposure. Using a well-ventilated area is key to maintaining a safe environment, especially when working with larger batches of soap.

Soap Molds: Choosing the Right One

As mentioned earlier, soap molds play a significant role in determining the final shape and appearance of your soap. The choice of mold will depend on the size, shape, and design you want for your soap bars. There are several types of molds to choose from, each with its own advantages and considerations:

1. Silicone Molds

Silicone molds are a favorite among soap makers because they are flexible and non-stick, allowing for easy removal of the soap once it has hardened. These molds come in various shapes and sizes, from simple rectangular bars to intricate designs like flowers, animals, or custom shapes. Silicone molds are also easy to clean and reuse, making them a practical option for hobbyists and small-batch soap makers.

2. Wooden Molds

Wooden molds are ideal for larger batches of soap and provide excellent insulation during the curing process. When lined with freezer paper or wax paper, the soap can be easily removed once it has hardened. The insulation offered by wooden molds helps retain heat, which can affect the texture and hardness of the soap. Wooden molds are typically used for rectangular loaves, which can be cut into individual bars once cured.

3. Plastic Molds

Plastic molds are less expensive than silicone or wooden options and are available in a wide range of designs. However, they are less flexible, making it more challenging to remove the soap without damaging the mold. For beginners, plastic molds can be a cost-effective way to experiment with different shapes before investing in higher-quality molds.

4. Homemade Molds

For the creative and resourceful soap maker, homemade molds are an excellent way to save money and add a personal touch to your products. Common household items like cardboard boxes, Tupperware containers, or even empty milk cartons can be lined with freezer paper and used as soap molds. These DIY molds are a great option for those looking to experiment without investing in expensive equipment.

Sourcing Equipment: Affordable Options

Building a soap-making toolkit doesn't have to be expensive. Many of the essential tools can be found in your kitchen or purchased secondhand. Here are a few tips for sourcing affordable equipment:

- Repurpose kitchen tools: Items like measuring cups, spatulas, and mixing bowls can often be repurposed for soap making, as long as they are kept separate from food preparation once used with lye.

- Thrift stores and online marketplaces: Secondhand stores and online marketplaces like eBay or Facebook Marketplace can be excellent sources for affordable molds, scales, and blenders.

- DIY solutions: As mentioned earlier, homemade molds are a cost-effective way to create custom shapes without spending a lot of money. Get creative with items you already have at home!

Maintenance and Care of Equipment

To ensure the longevity of your soap-making equipment, proper maintenance is essential. Here are some tips to keep your tools in good condition:

- Clean promptly: After each soap-making session, clean your equipment thoroughly to prevent soap residue from hardening. Use warm, soapy water and a sponge to scrub away any remaining soap batter.

- Store properly: Keep your equipment in a cool, dry place to prevent damage from moisture or heat. Silicone molds should be stored flat to avoid warping, while wooden molds should be stored in a well-ventilated area to prevent moisture buildup.

- Inspect regularly: Check your equipment regularly for any signs of wear and tear. Molds, in particular, should be inspected for cracks or warping, as this can affect the appearance and quality of your soap. Ensure your thermometers and scales are accurate by testing them periodically, and replace any equipment that shows signs of deterioration.

1. Deep Clean Periodically

In addition to routine cleaning after each use, it's also important to give your equipment a deep clean every so often. This is particularly important for items like your stick blender, which can accumulate oils in hard-to-reach places. Disassemble your stick blender (if possible) and soak the parts in warm, soapy water to dissolve any buildup.

Similarly, mixing containers, molds, and utensils may benefit from an occasional soak in a vinegar-water solution, which helps to neutralize any lingering lye residue. Rinse everything thoroughly afterward, and make sure all your tools are completely dry before storing them.

2. Dry Thoroughly

Moisture is one of the main enemies of soap-making equipment, particularly for metal tools like your scale or thermometer, as they can rust over time. After washing, dry your equipment thoroughly with a clean towel, and allow any remaining water to evaporate before putting your tools away.

If you live in a particularly humid area, consider using silica packets in your storage area to absorb excess moisture. Wooden molds especially need to be kept in a well-ventilated, dry area to prevent them from warping or developing mold.

3. Keep It Organized

Keeping your soap-making tools organized and in one designated area will make the process much smoother each time you begin a new batch. Use labeled containers or drawers to store your smaller items, such as thermometers and spatulas, and keep larger items like molds and mixing containers stacked neatly in a cupboard or shelf. Having everything in its place not only keeps your workspace tidy but also ensures that you can quickly find what you need when you're ready to start creating.

Conclusion

Proper equipment is the foundation of successful goat milk soap making. Each piece of equipment, from the digital scale to the molds, serves a critical purpose in the process. By investing in the right tools and taking good care of them, you'll not only ensure your soap batches turn out beautifully, but also create a safe and efficient workspace.

Remember, soap-making is both an art and a science. The tools you use will influence everything from the soap's texture and appearance to its safety and longevity. Whether you're just starting out or you're an experienced soap maker looking to improve your setup, understanding the role and maintenance of each tool will enhance your overall soap-making experience. Let's continue this journey into the world of natural, handmade beauty products.

Chapter Four:
The Soap-Making Process:
Cold Process vs Hot Process

When it comes to soap-making, the two most popular methods are the cold process and the hot process. Each has its own benefits and challenges, particularly when working with goat milk as a primary ingredient. Understanding these processes allows you to choose the method that best suits your needs, depending on your goals, equipment, and time.

This chapter will break down the cold and hot processes in detail, covering their pros and cons, the steps involved in each, and why the cold process is often favored for making goat milk soap. We'll also cover essential tips for working with lye safely, maintaining a controlled environment, and avoiding common beginner mistakes.

Overview of Cold Process vs. Hot Process Soap-Making

Both cold and hot processes require a combination of lye (sodium hydroxide), oils, and additional ingredients to produce soap. However, they differ significantly in terms of time, temperature, and how the final product cures. Let's explore each process in depth.

Cold Process Soap-Making

The cold process is one of the most traditional methods of soap-making. In this approach, the oils and lye are combined at room temperature or slightly warmed, which minimizes heat exposure. This method involves a chemical reaction called saponification, where the oils and lye mix to form soap.

Advantages of Cold Process:

1. Preserve Ingredients: Cold process soap preserves the natural qualities of goat milk and other ingredients, making it ideal for milk soaps.

2. Creamy Texture: Cold process soap often results in a smoother, creamier texture.

3. Longer Shelf Life: The cold process can enhance the shelf life of natural ingredients in the soap, giving it a stable structure and rich lather.

Disadvantages of the Cold Process:

1. Longer Cure Time: Cold process soap requires a curing period of 4-6 weeks to reach optimal hardness and mildness.

2. Milk Scorching: Because the cold process relies on room temperature, there's a risk of scorching the milk if the lye is too hot when added to the milk.

Hot Process Soap-Making

In the hot process soap-making, the mixture is heated to speed up saponification. This technique often involves using a slow cooker or stove to bring the soap to a gel-like consistency, which means the soap is closer to being fully saponified by the end of the process.

Advantages of Hot Process:

1. Faster Cure Time: Hot process soap is technically ready for use sooner and may only require a few days to a week of curing.

2. Textured Appearance: Hot process soap has a more rustic, textured appearance, which can be visually appealing.

Disadvantages of Hot Process:

1. Less Control Over Texture: Due to the thick, gel-like consistency, hot process soap can be harder to work with for those who prefer a smooth finish.

2. Heated Oils May Lose Properties: Heating can reduce the beneficial properties of some oils and additives.

3. Higher Risk of Milk Scorching: The high temperatures involved pose a risk of scorching the milk if the process is not carried out with utmost care.

Why Cold Process Is Preferred for Goat Milk Soap

For goat milk soap, the cold process is generally recommended due to its gentler approach, which preserves the nutrients in goat milk. Because goat milk contains sugars, proteins, and fats, it is prone to scorching when exposed to high heat. By keeping temperatures low in the cold process, you retain these valuable nutrients and ensure the milk doesn't caramelize, which would affect the soap's color and fragrance.

Step-by-Step Guide to Cold Process Soap-Making:

- Prepare Your Workspace: Set up your workspace with all the necessary equipment (molds, gloves, goggles, thermometer, etc.), and ensure it's well-ventilated.

- Prepare the Goat Milk: For cold process soap, it's recommended to freeze the goat milk in ice cube trays beforehand. Frozen milk helps to keep the temperature low, reducing the chance of scorching.

Combine the Lye and Goat Milk:

1. Wear protective gear: Put on gloves, goggles, and long sleeves to prevent lye burns.

2. Add lye to milk slowly: In a heatproof container, slowly add the lye to the frozen milk. Stir continuously as the lye melts the milk, maintaining a controlled reaction. The solution will heat up naturally, so go slowly to prevent a temperature spike.

3. Melt the Oils: In a separate container, gently melt your oils (such as coconut oil, olive oil, and palm oil) until they reach around 100°F (38°C).

4. Combine Oils and Lye Mixture: Once both the lye-milk solution and oils are at approximately the same temperature, slowly pour the lye solution into the oils. Blend with a stick blender until you achieve a thick consistency, known as "trace."

5. Add Essential Oils and Colorants (optional): Once you reach trace, you can add essential oils, colorants, or other additives.

6. Pour into Molds: Pour the mixture into soap molds, smooth the surface, and tap the mold gently to release any air bubbles.

7. Insulate and Cure: Cover the molds with a lid or plastic wrap, and let them sit in a cool, dark area for 24 hours. Afterward, remove the soap from the molds and let it cure for 4-6 weeks.

Step-by-Step Guide to Hot Process Soap-Making

1. Prepare Your Workspace: Gather your materials and set up a slow cooker or double boiler to heat the soap mixture.

2. Prepare the Lye and Goat Milk Solution: As with the cold process, use frozen goat milk and add the lye gradually to avoid scorching.

3. Melt the Oils: Add your oils to the slow cooker or pot and heat them gently until fully melted.

4. Combine Lye Solution and Oils: Pour the lye solution into the heated oils. Stir gently, then use a stick blender to bring the mixture to trace.

5. Cook the Soap Mixture: Set the slow cooker to a low setting. As the mixture heats, it will go through several stages:

6. Thick Trace: The mixture thickens and becomes gel-like.

7. Vaseline Stage: The soap develops a shiny, translucent appearance, indicating it's close to fully saponified.

8. Add Essential Oils and Colorants (optional): Once the soap reaches the Vaseline stage, you can add essential oils and colorants without the risk of evaporation.

9. Scoop into Molds: Scoop the thickened soap into molds, pressing it down to eliminate air pockets.

10. Cure for a Few Days: Although hot process soap can technically be used sooner, a brief curing period (about a week) allows it to harden further.

Safety Tips for Handling Lye

Working with lye requires caution. Here are essential safety practices:

- Wear Protective Gear: Always wear gloves, safety goggles, and long sleeves when handling lye.

- Ventilate: Work in a well-ventilated area or near an open window to avoid inhaling fumes.

- Add Lye to Liquid, Not Vice Versa: Pour the lye into the liquid slowly, never the other way around, to prevent splashes and intense reactions.

- Use Heatproof Containers: Only use containers specifically rated for heat and chemical resistance.

Common Mistakes in Cold Process and Hot Process Soap-Making

Cold Process Mistakes

- Overheating the Milk: If the lye is added too quickly to milk or not monitored carefully, it can cause scorching, affecting the soap's appearance and scent.

    o Solution: Use frozen goat milk and add the lye gradually, stirring continuously to keep the temperature steady.

- Inadequate Insulation: Cold process soap needs to saponify slowly over time. Failing to insulate the mold can result in uneven curing.

    o Solution: Cover your soap mold and place it in a cool, dark area for at least 24 hours before unmolding it.

- Not Reaching Proper Trace: Sometimes soap fails to reach a thick enough trace, which can cause the oils and lye to separate.

    o Solution: Use a stick blender to ensure the mixture reaches a proper trace. You're looking for a thick, pudding-like consistency.

Hot Process Mistakes

- Overheating: If the soap overheats, it can overflow from the slow cooker or pot.

  - Solution: Keep the heat on low and monitor the soap mixture. If it begins to bubble or rise too quickly, lower the heat or turn it off briefly.

- Uneven Consistency: Since hot process soap is thick, it can be challenging to get an even texture.

  - Solution: Stir thoroughly before pouring into molds, and tap the mold to release air bubbles.

- Inaccurate Temperatures: If the oils or lye solution are too hot or cold, the soap may not cook evenly.

  - Solution: Always monitor temperatures and aim for consistency, particularly when adding the lye solution.

In summary, both cold and hot processes offer distinct advantages for soap-making. The cold process is typically preferred for goat milk soap to preserve the milk's nutrients, though the hot process may be desirable for its shorter cure time and rustic texture. By following these detailed steps and safety guidelines, you'll be well-equipped to experiment with both techniques and create high-quality goat milk soap tailored to your preferences.

⤳

Chapter Five:
Understanding Oils, Lye, and Additives

Crafting high-quality goat milk soap involves understanding the fundamental ingredients and their roles in the soap-making process. In this chapter, we'll dive into the primary components: lye, oils, and additives. By understanding these elements, you'll be able to make informed decisions about how each ingredient affects your soap's texture, scent, lather, and moisturizing properties.

This chapter will cover why lye is a vital ingredient, the characteristics of common oils, the benefits of natural additives, and how to balance oils and additives to create a soap that meets your preferences.

The Role of Lye in Soap Making

Lye, or sodium hydroxide, is essential in traditional soap-making. While it may seem intimidating due to its caustic nature, lye is the ingredient that triggers saponification—the chemical reaction that turns oils and fats into soap.

Why Lye Is Necessary

Lye plays a critical role in soap-making because it breaks down the triglycerides in oils and combines with fatty acids to create soap molecules. Without lye, the oils would remain oils, and no soap would form. However, once the lye has fully reacted with the oils, it disappears, leaving no residual caustic substance in the finished product. This is why properly cured soap is safe for the skin, even though it begins with lye.

Key Tips for Working Safely with Lye

- Wear Protective Gear: Always use gloves, goggles, and long sleeves to avoid contact with lye.

- Use Heatproof, Non-Reactive Containers: Lye reacts strongly with some materials, so use containers made of heat-resistant plastic or glass.

- Add Lye to Liquids, Not Vice Versa: Always pour the lye into the liquid (such as goat milk) slowly, never the other way around, to avoid intense reactions and splashes. When using frozen cubes of goat milk, gently drop them in at an angle so they slide against the edge to prevent splashing lye around.

- Ventilation: Ensure you're in a well-ventilated area to avoid inhaling fumes when lye is dissolved.

Exploring Oils in Goat Milk Soap

The oils you choose in soap-making influence the final product's lather, hardness, moisturizing qualities, and cleansing properties. Each oil brings unique qualities, making understanding their characteristics and how they interact is essential.

Common Oils and Their Properties

1. Olive Oil

   - Properties: Olive oil is known for its gentle, moisturizing properties and is a staple in traditional soap-making, dating back centuries. It produces a creamy, mild lather that is especially beneficial for people with sensitive or dry skin.

   - Soap Qualities: Soap made with a high percentage of olive oil is highly conditioning, making it ideal for those seeking a nourishing and gentle product. However, soap made solely from olive oil, known as "Castile soap," can be softer and require longer curing times to achieve a firm bar. Often, it's blended with harder oils to strike a balance between conditioning and firmness.

   - Usage: Typically, olive oil constitutes 15-40% of the total oils in a recipe, allowing flexibility depending on desired conditioning and lather qualities.

2. Coconut Oil

   - Properties: Known for its versatility, coconut oil creates a hard, durable bar with a rich, bubbly lather. It has a high cleansing ability, making it effective for removing dirt and excess oils from the skin.

- Soap Qualities: Coconut oil adds a robust cleansing quality to soap. However, its strong cleansing action can be drying if used in high percentages. To counteract potential dryness, coconut oil is often balanced with conditioning oils such as olive or castor oil.

- Usage: Generally, coconut oil is used at 10-30% of the total oils in a recipe, depending on the desired level of lather and hardness. Keeping coconut oil within this range helps prevent skin dryness while enhancing the soap's durability.

3. Almond Oil

- Properties: Almond oil is valued for its lightweight, moisturizing qualities, contributing to a soft, creamy texture in soap. It creates a smooth, silky lather and adds a gentle touch, helping to produce a bar that is both nourishing and long-lasting.

- Soap Qualities: Almond oil provides a balance between the cleansing power of oils like coconut oil and the conditioning properties of softer oils. This makes it a great choice for achieving a well-rounded soap that lathers effectively while remaining mild on the skin.

- Usage: Almond oil is typically used in soap recipes at 20-30% of the total oils. Its combination of light texture, moisturizing properties, and ability to enhance the lather makes it a perfect complement to other oils, improving the overall feel and longevity of the soap.

4. Castor Oil

- Properties: Castor oil has a unique, thick texture that boosts lather and adds a silky feel to soap. It attracts and retains moisture, giving soap a luxurious feel when combined with other oils.

- Soap Qualities: While too soft to be used alone, castor oil excels at enhancing lather. It's particularly effective in recipes that need a creamy, stable foam without sacrificing conditioning.

- Usage: Castor oil is generally used at 5-10% of the recipe, as even small amounts significantly boost lather without softening the bar excessively.

5. Shea Butter

- Properties: Shea butter is rich in vitamins A and E, and is known for its skin-nourishing benefits. This butter adds a silky texture and extra moisturizing qualities to soap, making it ideal for dry or sensitive skin.

- Soap Qualities: While it doesn't contribute much to lather, shea butter enhances the conditioning properties of soap. It adds creaminess and soothes the skin, creating a bar that feels luxurious and gentle.

- Usage: Typically used at 5-15%, shea butter can soften the bar if used in large amounts, so it's often combined with harder oils to maintain firmness.

6. Tallow

- Properties: Tallow, rendered from beef fat, is a traditional soap-making ingredient known for its creamy lather and smooth texture. It imparts a "back-to-the-roots" feel, bringing old-fashioned quality to soap recipes. Rich in stearic and oleic acids, it's highly conditioning and adds longevity to bars.

- Soap Qualities: Tallow creates a hard bar with a stable, creamy lather, contributing to the soap's cleansing and conditioning properties. Its thick consistency makes for long-lasting bars that hold their shape well.

- Usage: Typically used at 20-50% of the recipe, tallow can act as a base for a well-rounded soap or be blended with other oils for added skin benefits.

7. Lard

- Properties: Lard, derived from pork fat, is another traditional soap-making fat with deep roots in homesteading and heritage recipes. It produces a mild, conditioning soap with a silky lather and leaves skin feeling soft without any greasy residue.

- Soap Qualities: Lard adds hardness and creaminess to soap, yielding bars that are firm yet gentle on the skin. The conditioning properties make it ideal for sensitive skin, while its economical nature makes it a sustainable choice for large batches.

- Usage: Often used at 20-50% in recipes, lard serves as a versatile base that pairs well with oils like coconut or castor to balance cleansing and lather qualities.

Blending Oils for Balanced Soap Qualities

When formulating a recipe, consider the following balance:

- Lather: Coconut and castor oils enhance lather, with coconut providing bubbles and castor creating a creamy foam.

- Conditioning: Olive oil, shea butter, and other soft oils enhance moisturizing properties.

- Hardness: Hard oils like coconut and palm create a firm bar that lasts longer.

Example Recipe Balance:

1. 30% Olive Oil (conditioning)

2. 25% Coconut Oil (lather and hardness)

3. 20% Palm Oil (hardness and stable lather)

4. 15% Shea Butter (conditioning)

5. 10% Castor Oil (lather booster)

Enhancing Your Soap with Natural Additives

Additives give soap personality and added benefits, from colors and scents to exfoliation and therapeutic properties.

Herbs and Botanicals

Herbs, such as lavender, chamomile, and rosemary, add a natural touch and can infuse soap with soothing or invigorating properties. Herbs can be used as dried petals for visual appeal or infused into oils before the soap-making process.

Clays and Mineral Additives

Clays such as kaolin, bentonite, and French green clay are popular in soap-making for their natural colors and detoxifying properties. Clays add a smooth, dense texture and are beneficial for oily or acne-prone skin as they help draw out impurities.

- Kaolin Clay: This mild, fine clay is gentle on the skin, making it suitable for all skin types, including sensitive and dry skin. Kaolin clay provides a soft, creamy lather and is ideal for adding a touch of silkiness to soap without stripping the skin of moisture.

- Bentonite Clay: Known for its impressive oil-absorbing properties, bentonite clay is derived from volcanic ash and works particularly well for oily and acne-prone skin. It creates a smooth, dense texture and gives soap a bit more "slip," which feels luxurious when applied to the skin. Bentonite is effective at drawing out toxins and impurities, making it a popular choice in detoxifying soaps.

- French Green Clay: This mineral-rich clay is celebrated for its natural green hue, adding a touch of color to soap without synthetic dyes. French green clay is excellent for detoxifying and toning the skin, as it absorbs oils and tightens pores, making it suitable for combination and oily skin types.

- Activated Charcoal: Activated charcoal is a highly porous substance renowned for its ability to deeply cleanse and purify the skin. It's incredibly effective at drawing out toxins, bacteria, and impurities, making it a popular choice for soaps aimed at oily or acne-prone skin. In addition to its detoxifying qualities, activated charcoal adds a striking black or gray color to soap, giving it a distinctive aesthetic. Small amounts can provide gentle exfoliation, while larger amounts create a more intense cleansing effect.

Exfoliants

Exfoliants help slough off dead skin cells, leaving the skin smoother and more radiant. Common natural exfoliants include:

- Oatmeal: Gentle and nourishing, oatmeal is ideal for sensitive and dry skin. It soothes irritation, reduces inflammation, and offers mild exfoliation, which makes it popular for sensitive skin and even baby soaps.

- Coffee Grounds: Coffee grounds provide a firmer exfoliating texture that's excellent for rough areas like elbows, knees, and feet. They can invigorate the skin, promote circulation, and add a natural brown speckling to the soap.

- Poppy Seeds: Offering a light, gentle exfoliation, poppy seeds add a unique visual appeal with small, dark specks in the soap. Suitable for all skin types, they work well in face and body soaps that need a mild scrubbing action.

Balancing Additives for Desired Effects

When adding exfoliants or herbs, moderation is key. Too much can cause the soap to become abrasive or not bind well. Typically, 1-2 tablespoons per pound of oils is a good starting point for exfoliants, while dried herbs are used in smaller amounts to avoid clumping.

Essential Oils for Scent and Therapeutic Benefits

Essential oils serve as natural fragrance agents and can provide therapeutic benefits through aromatherapy. For instance:

- Lavender: Known for its calming and soothing properties, lavender essential oil is ideal for evening soaps. It helps to relax the mind and can ease tension, making it a favorite in bedtime routines.

- Tea Tree: With natural antiseptic and antibacterial qualities, tea tree oil is excellent for acne-prone or oily skin. Its powerful purifying properties help cleanse the skin, making it suitable for face and body soaps targeting problem areas.

- Peppermint: Invigorating and refreshing, peppermint essential oil adds a gentle cooling sensation that revitalizes the skin and awakens the senses. Its natural menthol content is perfect for morning showers, promoting alertness and freshness.

Tips for Using Essential Oils

- Dosage: Essential oils are potent, so a general rule is to use around 0.5-1 ounce of essential oil per pound of oils in your soap.

- Blending: Consider combining essential oils for a more complex fragrance. For example, lavender and eucalyptus make a relaxing blend, while lemon and peppermint create an uplifting scent.

Balancing Oils and Additives for Desired Soap Qualities

Achieving the right balance of oils, lye, and additives takes practice and experimentation. Here's a quick guide:

1. Define Your Goals: Determine whether you want a moisturizing bar, a firm soap that lasts long, or a highly cleansing bar. This will help you prioritize the types of oils to use.

2. Adjust for Hardness and Lather: Use a combination of hard and soft oils to ensure the bar maintains structure and creates a good lather.

3. Additives for Function and Aesthetics: Choose additives that align with your soap's purpose. For example, clays and exfoliants work well for a cleansing bar, while herbs and butters add nourishment.

4. Measure Carefully: Use a digital scale to ensure precision. Even small variations in oil-to-lye ratios can impact the soap's quality and safety.

Crafting high-quality goat milk soap involves a careful selection of lye, oils, and additives to achieve your desired soap qualities. By understanding the role of each component, you'll be equipped to create a product that is both functional and enjoyable to use.

~∽

Chapter Six:
How to Make Goat Milk Soap

Goat milk soap offers a gentle, nourishing cleanse for the skin. It is packed with natural fats, vitamins, and minerals that provide a soothing lather. This chapter provides a thorough, step-by-step guide to making goat milk soap from scratch, ensuring you can create a bar that maintains the beneficial properties of goat milk while achieving the ideal consistency and quality.

Step-by-Step Guide to Making Goat Milk Soap

Making goat milk soap involves precise measurements, proper preparation, and an understanding of each step in the process. The following instructions will guide you through creating a batch of goat milk soap, whether you're a beginner or an experienced soap maker.

1. Gathering Ingredients and Equipment

Ingredients:

- Goat milk (chilled or frozen to prevent scorching)

- Sodium hydroxide (lye)

- Oils and butters (e.g., olive oil, coconut oil, shea butter, etc.)

- Essential oils (optional for scent)

- Natural additives (optional for color and texture)

Equipment:

- Safety gear (goggles, gloves, apron)

- Digital kitchen scale for precise measurement

- Heat-safe containers (preferably heavy plastic for lye and milk mixture)

- Stick blender to achieve proper trace

- Soap molds

- Thermometer to monitor temperature

- Spatula, spoons, and a mixing bowl

2. Safety First

Working with lye requires careful handling to avoid burns or respiratory irritation:

- Wear protective gear: Use goggles, gloves, and a long-sleeved shirt to protect your skin and eyes from lye splashes.

- Work in a ventilated area: Always make soap in a well-ventilated space or near an open window, as the lye mixture emits fumes when combined with liquids.

- Add lye to liquids, not vice versa: Slowly add lye to goat milk (or water if dissolving lye separately) to prevent splashing and excessive heat buildup.

3. Measuring and Preparing Ingredients

Accurate measurements are essential for achieving a high-quality bar of soap, as even small deviations can affect the texture, hardness, and overall performance of your soap.

Weighing Each Ingredient Precisely:

- Using a digital kitchen scale is highly recommended, as it allows you to measure each ingredient with precision, down to the gram. This accuracy is particularly important when handling lye, which must be balanced exactly with the oils to ensure complete saponification.

- Double-check your recipe and measurements before beginning, especially if you're adjusting batch sizes. Even a small discrepancy in the amount of lye or liquid can cause the soap to be either too harsh (if there's too much lye) or too soft (if there's too little).

- Keep a soap-making journal to record measurements, oil types, and any adjustments you make. This practice is especially helpful for identifying patterns in the soap's texture, lather, or hardness if you're experimenting with different formulas.

Preparing the Goat Milk:

- Goat milk brings beneficial properties to the soap, but it's also sensitive to temperature. To protect its natural fats, vitamins, and proteins, chill or freeze the goat milk before mixing with lye. Frozen or partially frozen milk helps prevent excessive heat that can lead to discoloration, curdling, or scorching.

- If possible, freeze the goat milk in ice cube trays for easy handling and to slow down the rise in temperature as lye is added. Smaller cubes melt more gradually, allowing better control during the mixing process.

- Additionally, keeping the goat milk cold preserves its creamy color and nutrient content, which contributes to the soap's mildness and luxurious feel.

Setting Up a Clean, Organized Workspace:

- Arrange your ingredients and tools within easy reach to maintain a smooth workflow during soap-making. Lye should be kept in a separate container to prevent accidental spills, and oils should be measured and ready to melt before beginning.

- Since soap-making requires precision, take time to double-check your supplies, making sure everything is prepared and sanitized. This approach reduces interruptions and makes it easier to handle the steps in sequence, especially when working with temperature-sensitive ingredients like goat milk.

By focusing on careful measurements and preparation, you ensure that each ingredient performs its function in the final soap bar, from the nourishing qualities of goat milk to the specific roles of different oils. This attention to detail contributes to a consistent and successful soap-making experience.

Tip: *To maintain the creamy color and properties of goat milk, gradually incorporate lye while stirring the mixture to avoid curdling.*

4. Creating the Lye and Goat Milk Mixture

For goat milk soap, the lye solution is a critical step in preserving the milk's benefits:

1. Slowly add lye to frozen or chilled goat milk in a heat-resistant container, stirring constantly. This gradual process will control temperature and prevent the milk from scorching.

2. Stir until the lye is fully dissolved, with a smooth, uniform consistency.

Tip: *Goat milk's sugars can cause the mixture to darken or discolor if heated too quickly, so patience is key.*

5. Heating and Mixing Oils

Once your lye and milk mixture is ready, melt and combine oils:

1. Heat oils and butters in a separate container until fully melted. If using solid butters like shea or cocoa butter,

melt them before adding liquid oils, like olive or coconut oil.

2. Allow oils to cool to around 100-110°F before mixing with the lye solution to reduce the risk of uneven saponification.

Tip: Matching the temperature of the oils and lye solution helps achieve a more even trace.

6. Combining Lye Solution and Oils

This step initiates the chemical reaction, known as saponification, which transforms the fats and lye into soap. Proceed slowly and carefully, as combining these ingredients requires attention to both technique and timing.

Pouring the Lye and Goat Milk Solution into the Oils:

Gently and steadily pour the lye and chilled goat milk solution into the warmed oils, stirring continuously with a spatula to ensure even distribution. Pouring slowly prevents sudden temperature shifts that could cause splattering or affect the soap's texture.

Using a heavy plastic or heat-resistant glass container for mixing is recommended, as these materials are less likely to react with lye.

Blending to Reach "Trace:"

With a stick blender set to low speed, pulse and stir the mixture in short bursts, alternating with manual stirring to prevent over-blending. Trace is reached when the soap mixture thickens to a pudding-like consistency, leaving visible trails or "traces" when dripped from the blender. Reaching trace indicates the oils and lye have begun bonding, marking the start of the saponification process.

Trace can occur quickly or take several minutes, depending on the oils used and the ambient temperature, so watch closely to avoid over-thickening.

Incorporating Essential Oils and Additives:

At this stage, add any essential oils, colorants, or exfoliants you've chosen, stirring gently to incorporate them evenly. Essential oils can evaporate if over-mixed, so fold them lightly with the stick blender or a spatula.

Ensuring even distribution of additives at trace locks in scent, color, and therapeutic benefits, creating a balanced and high-quality soap.

Taking these steps with care preserves the qualities of your ingredients and ensures a smooth, consistent soap texture in the final product.

7. Achieving the Ideal Consistency and Pouring into Molds

Trace is a vital stage in soap-making that determines texture and hardness:

- Thin trace is fluid, ideal for swirling designs; medium trace holds a slight texture; thick trace is ready for solid designs or exfoliants.

- Once the mixture reaches the desired consistency, pour into molds evenly, tapping the mold gently to remove air bubbles.

Tip: *Smooth the surface with a spatula for a polished look,*
or add decorative textures if desired.

8. Curing and Storing Soap

Proper curing is crucial to creating a stable, high-quality bar:

1. After pouring, cover the soap molds and wrap them in a towel or blanket to insulate for 24 hours. Insulating helps the soap go through the gel phase, enhancing color and texture. Can put wax paper between the towel and soap.

2. After 24 hours, unmold the soap and slice it into bars, then place bars on a rack to cure for 4-6 weeks. This curing time allows the soap to harden, enhancing longevity and lather.

Tip: *Store soap in a cool, dry place away from direct sunlight to*
prevent discoloration or warping.

Tips for Incorporating Goat Milk Successfully

Adding goat milk to soap can be tricky, but with a few careful steps, you can maintain its benefits without compromising quality:

1. Chill or freeze milk beforehand: Freezing reduces the risk of burning or curdling.

2. Add lye gradually: Stir continuously while adding lye to avoid rapid temperature increases.

3. Monitor color: If the milk turns too brown or orange, it may have scorched, so consider starting with partially frozen milk for better control.

Troubleshooting Common Issues

Soap-making requires careful attention to detail, as small deviations in temperature, mixing, or measurements can impact the final product. Here are some of the most common issues encountered in goat milk soap-making, along with solutions to help you troubleshoot and refine your process.

1. Curdling

   - Issue: The goat milk and lye mixture curdles, appearing clumpy or separating.

   - Cause: Curdling typically happens when the lye solution is too hot, which can scorch the milk proteins, leading to curdling.

   - Solution: To avoid curdling, use partially frozen or well-chilled goat milk and add the lye gradually, stirring constantly to prevent temperature spikes. Adding lye too quickly can heat the mixture rapidly, so pour it slowly and blend carefully.

2. Improper Trace

   - Issue: The mixture either reaches the trace too soon or the trace appears uneven.

   - Cause: Trace, the point at which the soap batter thickens to a pudding-like texture, can be impacted by excessive or inconsistent blending.

   - Solution: Use short bursts with a stick blender, interspersed with manual stirring. This helps control the speed at which trace develops and ensures all ingredients are well incorporated. Avoid continuous blending, which can accelerate trace unexpectedly, making the mixture hard to work with.

3. Air Bubbles

- Issue: Visible bubbles or pockets form in the finished soap, affecting its appearance.

- Cause: Air bubbles typically arise from over-blending or not releasing trapped air before setting.

- Solution: Once the soap mixture is poured into the mold, tap the mold firmly on the counter several times to release the trapped air. This simple step helps create a smoother texture by eliminating air pockets.

4. Soft Soap

- Issue: Soap feels overly soft or mushy, even after curing.

- Cause: Excess liquid or high humidity can contribute to a softer texture. Using too much water in the lye solution or oils with a high moisture content can also cause this issue.

- Solution: Extend the curing time by a few weeks to allow more water to evaporate, which will help the soap harden. Alternatively, consider adjusting your recipe by reducing water content slightly or adding harder oils like coconut or palm oil.

5. Crumbly Texture

- Issue: Soap crumbles or breaks easily when cut or unmolded.

- Cause: Overuse of lye or excessive heat during saponification can result in a brittle, crumbly texture.

- Solution: Double-check lye measurements with a digital scale to ensure accuracy. If crumbling persists, lower the heat by soaping at a slightly lower temperature or check that your oils are not overheated before combining them with the lye solution.

6. Separation of Oil and Lye

- Issue: Oils and lye refuse to combine, leaving an oily layer on top or visibly separated ingredients.

- Cause: Temperature differences between the lye solution and oils can prevent emulsification.

- Solution: Ensure both the lye solution and oils are within 10-15°F of each other before blending. This will encourage smooth blending and help achieve a stable emulsion. Use a thermometer to check the temperatures and warm or cool the ingredients to match.

Ideal Curing and Storage Techniques

The curing process transforms freshly made soap into a firm, long-lasting bar:

1. Spacing and Airflow: Place bars on a curing rack with space between each bar to allow air circulation, preventing dampness.

2. Monitoring Soap: Turn bars weekly for even drying, and check for any signs of excess moisture.

3. Duration: A minimum of 4-6 weeks is recommended, but some soap makers cure their bars for several months to achieve a superior bar that lasts longer and lathers richly.

Storing your soap after curing is equally important. Use breathable containers like cardboard boxes or wooden crates to store cured soap, avoiding plastic that could trap moisture.

This chapter equips you with every step necessary to create high-quality goat milk soap with confidence and consistency, from handling delicate goat milk to troubleshooting the most common soap-making challenges. With practice and attention to detail, you'll be able to make luxurious, creamy bars that nourish the skin and highlight the unique benefits of goat milk.

Chapter Seven:
Goat Milk Soap Recipes and How to Create
Your Own Recipes

Goat milk soap has earned its reputation as a beloved choice among natural skincare enthusiasts, thanks to its impressive array of skin benefits. Packed with natural emollients, vitamins, and triglycerides, goat milk works to soothe, moisturize, and rejuvenate sensitive, dry, and combination skin. Its creamy texture provides a gentle cleansing experience, making it particularly advantageous for those with sensitive skin, as it cleanses without stripping away the skin's essential oils. Additionally, goat milk is abundant in lactic acid, an alpha hydroxy acid (AHA) that facilitates the gentle exfoliation of dead skin cells, resulting in a smoother and more radiant complexion.

Soap-making transcends mere crafting; it is an art form that invites endless creativity and personalization. The process begins with the careful combination of oils, lye, and goat milk to form a luxurious base, which can then be customized with various additives, colors, and scents to reflect individual preferences. This creative freedom encourages experimentation, empowering soap makers to tailor their creations to meet specific skin needs or aesthetic aspirations. Whether you're designing a simple bar for daily use or an elaborate gift adorned with decorative embellishments, the possibilities are truly limitless.

One of the most enticing aspects of crafting your own goat milk soap is the ability to customize recipes to suit your unique skin requirements. For example, those with dry skin may choose to add nourishing ingredients like honey or oatmeal for enhanced moisture and gentle exfoliation. Conversely, individuals with oily skin might opt for purifying additives, such as activated charcoal or tea tree oil. Utilizing a soap calculator, like SoapCalc, allows soap makers to precisely adjust the ratios of oils and other ingredients, achieving the desired texture, hardness, and lather, ensuring that each bar is perfectly crafted for its intended purpose.

Making goat milk soap is a fulfilling and versatile craft that harmoniously blends the benefits of natural ingredients with the joy of creative expression. Whether you are a novice eager to explore the art of soap making or a seasoned artisan looking to refine your skills, the ability to customize and experiment with diverse recipes ensures that this engaging hobby will never lose its charm. Dive into the world of goat milk soap making and discover the endless possibilities that await!

Section 1: Basic Goat Milk Soap Recipes

Recipe 1: Classic Goat Milk Soap

Ingredients:

- 16 oz. (1 lb.) goat milk (frozen)

- 6 oz. lye (sodium hydroxide)

- 32 oz. (2 lb.) olive oil

- 16 oz. (1 lb.) coconut oil

- 16 oz. (1 lb.) almond oil

Optional: Essential oils for fragrance (e.g., lavender, eucalyptus)

Step-by-Step Instructions:

1. Prepare Your Workspace: Ensure your workspace is clean and well-ventilated. Gather all your ingredients and tools, including a digital scale, mixing bowls, a stick blender, a thermometer, and a soap mold.

2. Freeze the Goat Milk: To prevent the goat milk from scorching when mixed with lye, freeze it in ice cube trays until solid.

3. Mix the Lye Solution: In a well-ventilated area, carefully measure the lye using a digital scale. Slowly add the lye to the frozen goat milk (never the other way around) while stirring gently. The mixture will heat up and turn into a liquid. Allow it to cool to around 100-110°F (38-43°C).

4. Melt the Oils: In a separate pot, combine the olive oil, coconut oil, and almond oil. Heat gently until all oils are melted and combined. Allow the oils to cool to about 100-110°F (38-43°C).

5. Combine Lye and Oils: Once both the lye solution and oils are at the same temperature, slowly pour the lye solution into the oils while blending with a stick blender. Blend until you

reach "trace," which is when the mixture thickens and leaves a trail on the surface.

6. Add Optional Ingredients: If desired, add essential oils for fragrance and mix thoroughly.

7. Pour into Mold: Carefully pour the soap mixture into your mold, smoothing the top with a spatula. Cover the mold with a towel to insulate it.

8. Cure the Soap: Allow the soap to sit in the mold for 24-48 hours until it hardens. Once solid, remove it from the mold and cut it into bars.

9. Cure the Bars: Place the bars on a drying rack in a cool, dry area for 4-6 weeks to cure. This allows the soap to harden and the lye to fully saponify.

Tips for Beginners on Handling Lye Safely

- Wear Protective Gear: Always wear gloves, goggles, and long sleeves when handling lye to protect your skin and eyes from burns.

- Work in a Ventilated Area: Lye can produce fumes when mixed with liquids, so ensure your workspace is well-ventilated.

- Use Accurate Measurements: Always measure lye and liquids accurately using a digital scale to ensure safety and proper saponification.

- Store Lye Safely: Keep lye in a secure, labeled container away from children and pets.

Common Troubleshooting Tips for First-Time Soap Makers

- Soap is Too Soft: If your soap remains soft after the curing period, it may need more time to harden. Ensure you followed the recipe accurately, especially the lye-to-oil ratio.

- Lye Burns or Irritation: If you experience skin irritation, ensure you are wearing protective gear and working in a well-ventilated area. Always handle lye with care.

- Soap Has a Grainy Texture: This can occur if the oils were too hot when mixed with the lye. Ensure both the lye solution and oils are at similar temperatures before combining.

- Soap Fails to Trace: If your soap mixture doesn't thicken after blending, it may be due to incorrect measurements or temperatures. Double-check your ingredients and try again.

By following this classic goat milk soap recipe and these helpful tips, you'll be well on your way to creating beautiful, nourishing soap that your skin will love! Enjoy the process and embrace the creativity that comes with soap making.

Section 2: Herbal Goat Milk Soap Recipes

Recipe 2: Lavender and Chamomile Soap

Ingredients:

- 16 oz. (1 lb.) goat milk (frozen)

- 6 oz. lye (sodium hydroxide)

- 32 oz. (2 lb.) olive oil

- 16 oz. (1 lb.) coconut oil

- 16 oz. (1 lb.) almond oil

- 2 tablespoons dried lavender flowers

- 2 tablespoons dried chamomile flowers

- 1 oz. lavender essential oil

- Optional: Additional dried herbs for decoration

Detailed Instructions:

1. Prepare Your Workspace: As with any soap-making process, ensure your workspace is clean and well-ventilated. Gather all your ingredients and tools, including a digital scale, mixing bowls, a stick blender, a thermometer, and a soap mold.

2. Infuse the Oils with Herbs: To infuse the olive oil with the herbal properties of lavender and chamomile, combine the dried herbs with the olive oil in a small saucepan. Heat the mixture gently over low heat for about 30 minutes, ensuring it does not boil. This process allows the oils to extract the beneficial properties of the herbs. After infusing, strain the oil to remove the herbs and set it aside to cool. Alternatively, you can cold infuse the herbs in the oil but this is much more time consuming as it needs months instead of minutes to infuse.

3. Freeze the Goat Milk: Freeze the goat milk in ice cube trays until solid. This step helps prevent the milk from scorching when mixed with lye.

4. Mix the Lye Solution: In a well-ventilated area, carefully measure the lye using a digital scale. Slowly add the lye to the frozen goat milk while stirring gently. The mixture will heat up and turn into a liquid. Allow it to cool to around 100-110°F (38-43°C).

5. Melt the Oils: In a separate pot, combine the infused olive oil, coconut oil, and almond oil. Heat gently until all oils are melted and combined. Allow the oils to cool to about 100-110°F (38-43°C).

6. Combine Lye and Oils: Once both the lye solution and oils are at the same temperature, slowly pour the lye solution into the oils while blending with a stick blender. Blend until you reach "trace," which is when the mixture thickens and leaves a trail on the surface.

7. Add Essential Oils and Herbs: At trace, add the lavender essential oil and mix thoroughly. If desired, you can also add a small amount of the dried lavender and chamomile flowers to the soap mixture for added texture and visual appeal.

8. Pour into Mold: Carefully pour the soap mixture into your mold, smoothing the top with a spatula. Optionally, sprinkle some additional dried herbs on top for decoration.

9. Cure the Soap: Cover the mold with a towel to insulate it and allow the soap to sit for 24-48 hours until it hardens. Once solid, remove it from the mold and cut it into bars.

10. Cure the Bars: Place the bars on a drying rack in a cool, dry area for 4-6 weeks to cure. This allows the soap to harden and the lye to fully saponify.

Benefits of Using Essential Oils and Dried Herbs

Using essential oils and dried herbs in your soap not only enhances the fragrance but also provides additional skin benefits. Lavender essential oil is known for its calming and soothing properties, making it ideal for relaxation and stress relief. It can also help with minor skin irritations. Chamomile is renowned for its anti-inflammatory and soothing effects, making it perfect for sensitive skin. The inclusion of dried herbs adds texture and visual appeal, creating a more luxurious and artisanal product.

Variations with Other Herbal Combinations

Feel free to experiment with different herbal combinations to create unique soap recipes tailored to your preferences. Here are a few ideas:

- Rosemary and Mint: Infuse olive oil with dried rosemary and add peppermint essential oil for a refreshing, invigorating soap.

- Calendula and Tea Tree: Use calendula petals for their soothing properties and add tea tree oil for its antibacterial benefits, which are perfect for acne-prone skin.

- Eucalyptus and lemongrass: Combine eucalyptus leaves with lemongrass essential oil for a revitalizing and uplifting scent.

By infusing your goat milk soap with various herbs and essential oils, you can create a range of delightful and beneficial products that cater to different skin types and preferences. Enjoy the process of crafting your herbal goat milk soap, and let your creativity shine!

Recipe 3: Rosemary and Mint Soap

Ingredients:

- 16 oz. (1 lb.) goat milk (frozen)

- 6 oz. lye (sodium hydroxide)

- 32 oz. (2 lb.) olive oil

- 16 oz. (1 lb.) coconut oil

- 16 oz. (1 lb.) almond oil

- 1 oz. rosemary essential oil

- 0.75 oz. peppermint essential oil

Optional: Dried rosemary and mint for decoration

Preparation Steps:

1. Prepare Your Workspace: Ensure your workspace is clean and well-ventilated. Gather all necessary tools and ingredients, including a digital scale, mixing bowls, a stick blender, a thermometer, and a soap mold.

2. Freeze the Goat Milk: Freeze the goat milk in ice cube trays until solid. This helps prevent scorching when mixed with lye.

3. Mix the Lye Solution: In a well-ventilated area, carefully measure the lye using a digital scale. Slowly add the lye to the frozen goat milk while stirring gently. The mixture will heat up and turn into a liquid. Allow it to cool to around 100-110°F (38-43°C).

4. Melt the Oils: In a separate pot, combine the olive oil, coconut oil, and almond oil. Heat gently until all oils are melted and combined. Allow the oils to cool to about 100-110°F (38-43°C).

5. Combine Lye and Oils: Once both the lye solution and oils are at the same temperature, slowly pour the lye solution into the oils while blending with a stick blender. Blend until you reach "trace," which is when the mixture thickens and leaves a trail on the surface.

6. Add Essential Oils: At trace, add the rosemary and peppermint essential oils. Mix thoroughly to ensure the oils are evenly distributed throughout the soap mixture.

7. Pour into Mold: Carefully pour the soap mixture into your mold, smoothing the top with a spatula. If desired, sprinkle some dried rosemary and mint on top for added texture and decoration.

8. Cure the Soap: Cover the mold with a towel to insulate it and allow the soap to sit for 24-48 hours until it hardens. Once solid, remove it from the mold and cut it into bars.

9. Cure the Bars: Place the bars on a drying rack in a cool, dry area for 4-6 weeks to cure. This allows the soap to harden and the lye to fully saponify.

Discussion on the Invigorating Effects of Mint and Rosemary

The combination of rosemary and mint in this soap recipe not only creates a refreshing scent but also offers invigorating effects for the mind and body. Rosemary is known for its stimulating properties, often used to enhance mental clarity and focus. It can help alleviate fatigue and improve concentration, making it an excellent choice for morning showers or whenever you need a mental boost.

Mint, particularly peppermint, is renowned for its cooling and refreshing qualities. It can help awaken the senses and provide a burst of energy, making it perfect for revitalizing your skin and spirit. The combination of these two herbs creates a harmonious blend that can uplift your mood and invigorate your bathing experience.

How to Achieve Optimal Scent Balance

To achieve the perfect scent balance in your rosemary and mint soap, consider the following tips:

- Essential Oil Ratios: The suggested ratio of 1 oz rosemary essential oil to 0.75 oz peppermint essential oil provides a balanced fragrance. Rosemary has a stronger, more earthy scent, while peppermint is bright and refreshing. Adjusting these ratios can help you find your preferred scent profile. For a more robust mint scent, you can increase the peppermint slightly, but be cautious not to overpower the rosemary.

- Quality of Essential Oils: Use high-quality, pure essential oils for the best fragrance and therapeutic benefits. Synthetic fragrances may not provide the same invigorating effects and can sometimes irritate the skin.

- Testing Small Batches: If you're unsure about the scent balance, consider making a small test batch first. This allows you to experiment with different ratios without committing to a full batch.

- Add Dried Herbs: Incorporating dried rosemary and mint into the soap not only enhances the visual appeal but also adds a subtle herbal scent that complements the essential oils.

Following these guidelines, you can create a beautifully scented rosemary and mint soap that invigorates the senses and enhances your bathing experience. Enjoy the process of crafting this refreshing soap and the delightful benefits it brings!

Section 3: Exfoliating Goat Milk Soap Recipes

Recipe 4: Oatmeal and Honey Exfoliating Soap

Ingredients:

- 16 oz. (1 lb.) goat milk (frozen)

- 6 oz. lye (sodium hydroxide)

- 32 oz. (2 lb.) olive oil

- 16 oz. (1 lb.) coconut oil

- 16 oz. (1 lb.) almond oil

- 1 cup finely ground oatmeal (or rolled oats)

- 4 oz. honey

Optional: Additional oatmeal for decoration

Step-by-Step Guide:

1. Prepare Your Workspace: Ensure your workspace is clean and well-ventilated. Gather all necessary tools and ingredients, including a digital scale, mixing bowls, a stick blender, a thermometer, and a soap mold.

2. Freeze the Goat Milk: Freeze the goat milk in ice cube trays until solid. This helps prevent scorching when mixed with lye.

3. Mix the Lye Solution: In a well-ventilated area, carefully measure the lye using a digital scale. Slowly add the lye to the frozen goat milk while stirring gently. The mixture will heat up and turn into a liquid. Allow it to cool to around 100-110°F (38-43°C).

4. Melt the Oils: In a separate pot, combine the olive oil, coconut oil, and almond oil. Heat gently until all oils are melted and combined. Allow the oils to cool to about 100-110°F (38-43°C).

5. Combine Lye and Oils: Once both the lye solution and oils are at the same temperature, slowly pour the lye solution into the oils while blending with a stick blender. Blend until you reach "trace," which is when the mixture thickens and leaves a trail on the surface.

6. Add Oatmeal and Honey: At trace, add the finely ground oatmeal and honey to the soap mixture. Mix thoroughly to ensure even distribution. If desired, reserve some oatmeal for decoration.

7. Pour into Mold: Carefully pour the soap mixture into your mold, smoothing the top with a spatula. If using, sprinkle additional oatmeal on top for decoration.

8. Cure the Soap: Cover the mold with a towel to insulate it and allow the soap to sit for 24-48 hours until it hardens. Once solid, remove it from the mold and cut it into bars.

9. Cure the Bars: Place the bars on a drying rack in a cool, dry area for 4-6 weeks to cure. This allows the soap to harden and the lye to fully saponify.

The Dual Benefits of Honey as a Moisturizer and Healer

Honey is a remarkable ingredient in soap making, offering dual benefits for the skin. As a moisturizer, honey helps to attract and retain moisture, making it ideal for dry skin. Its humectant properties ensure that your skin feels hydrated and soft after use. Additionally, honey is known for its healing properties; it has natural antibacterial and anti-inflammatory effects, which can help soothe irritated skin and promote healing. This makes oatmeal and honey soap particularly beneficial for those with sensitive or troubled skin.

Adjusting Exfoliant Levels for Different Preferences

When it comes to exfoliation, personal preference plays a significant role. Here are some tips for adjusting the exfoliant levels in your oatmeal and honey soap:

- For Gentle Exfoliation: Use finely ground oatmeal, which provides a mild exfoliating effect suitable for sensitive skin. You can start with ½ cup of oatmeal and adjust based on your preference.

- For Moderate Exfoliation: If you prefer a more noticeable exfoliating effect, you can increase the amount of oatmeal to 1 cup. This will provide a more textured feel without being too harsh.

- For Stronger Exfoliation: Consider adding additional exfoliants, such as ground coffee or sugar, in small amounts. However, be cautious not to overwhelm the soap with too many exfoliants, as this can irritate the skin.

Recipe 5: Coffee Grounds and Sea Salt Soap

Ingredients:

- 16 oz. (1 lb.) goat milk (frozen)

- 6 oz. lye (sodium hydroxide)

- 32 oz. (2 lb.) olive oil

- 16 oz. (1 lb.) coconut oil

- 16 oz. (1 lb.) almond oil

- 1 cup used coffee grounds (cooled)

- ½ cup sea salt (fine or coarse)

Optional: Coffee essential oil for fragrance

Instructions for Incorporating Coffee Grounds and Sea Salt:

1. Prepare Your Workspace: As always, ensure your workspace is clean and well-ventilated. Gather all necessary tools and ingredients.

2. Freeze the Goat Milk: Freeze the goat milk in ice cube trays until solid.

3. Mix the Lye Solution: In a well-ventilated area, carefully measure the lye. Slowly add the lye to the frozen goat milk while stirring gently. Allow it to cool to around 100-110°F (38-43°C).

4. Melt the Oils: In a separate pot, combine the olive oil, coconut oil, and almond oil. Heat gently until melted and combined. Allow to cool to about 100-110°F (38-43°C).

5. Combine Lye and Oils: Once both the lye solution and oils are at the same temperature, slowly pour the lye solution into the oils while blending with a stick blender until you reach trace.

6. Add Coffee Grounds and Sea Salt: At trace, add the used coffee grounds and sea salt to the soap mixture. If desired, add a few drops of coffee essential oil for an extra boost of fragrance. Mix thoroughly to ensure even distribution.

7. Pour into Mold: Carefully pour the soap mixture into your mold, smoothing the top with a spatula.

8. Cure the Soap: Cover the mold with a towel and allow it to sit for 24-48 hours until hardened. Remove from the mold and cut into bars.

9. Cure the Bars: Place the bars on a drying rack in a cool, dry area for 4-6 weeks to cure.

Advantages of Using Natural Exfoliants

Using natural exfoliants like coffee grounds and sea salt in your soap offers several advantages:

- Gentle on the Skin: Natural exfoliants are often less abrasive than synthetic options, making them suitable for various skin types.

- Nourishing Properties: Coffee grounds contain antioxidants that can help protect the skin, while sea salt is rich in minerals that can nourish and revitalize.

- Sustainable and Eco-Friendly: Using coffee grounds, especially from your morning brew, promotes sustainability by repurposing waste materials.

Suggestions for Customizing Exfoliation Intensity

To customize the intensity of exfoliation in your coffee grounds and sea salt soap, consider the following:

- Adjusting Coffee Grounds: For a more intense exfoliation, increase the amount of coffee grounds. However, be mindful that too much can make the soap gritty.

- Choosing Sea Salt Texture: Fine Sea salt provides a gentler exfoliation, while coarse sea salt offers a more vigorous scrubbing effect. Choose based on your skin's sensitivity and your personal preference.

- Combining Exfoliants: Feel free to mix different exfoliants, such as adding oatmeal or sugar, to create a unique texture and exfoliation experience.

By following these recipes and tips, you can create exfoliating goat milk soaps that not only cleanse but also nourish and rejuvenate your skin. Enjoy the process of crafting these delightful soaps and the benefits they bring!

Section 4: Customizing Recipes with a Soap Calculator

Introduction to SoapCalc and Its Benefits

SoapCalc is an invaluable tool for soap makers, allowing you to create customized soap recipes with precision. This online lye calculator helps you determine the exact amounts of lye and oils needed for your soap, ensuring that your creations are safe and effective. By using SoapCalc, you can experiment with different oils, adjust ratios, and achieve the desired properties in your soap, such as hardness, lather, and moisturizing qualities. The benefits of using a soap calculator include:

1. Accuracy: Ensures the correct lye-to-oil ratio, preventing issues like lye-heavy soap.

2. Customization: Allows you to tailor recipes to your preferences, whether you want a specific scent, texture, or skin benefit.

3. Safety: Helps maintain proper pH levels in your soap, making it safe for use on the skin.

Detailed Instructions on Using a Soap Calculator

Understanding Lye Calculators and Saponification Values:

- Saponification Value: Each oil has a specific saponification value, which indicates how much lye is needed to convert a

72

given weight of that oil into soap. When using SoapCalc, you'll input the types and amounts of oils you plan to use, and the calculator will automatically determine the required amount of lye.

- Inputting Oils: Start by selecting the oils you want to use from the provided list. Enter the weight of each oil in ounces or grams. The calculator will display the total weight of oils and the corresponding lye amount needed.

Adjusting Oil Combinations and Ratios:

- Experimenting with Oils: You can mix and match different oils to achieve various properties in your soap. For example, adding coconut oil can increase lather, while olive oil can enhance moisturizing qualities.

- Adjusting Ratios: If you want a harder soap, increase the amount of almond oil or coconut oil. For a creamier lather, consider adding more olive oil. The calculator will update the lye amount based on your adjustments, ensuring you maintain the correct balance.

Ensuring Proper pH Balance and Curing Times:

- Superfatting: This is the practice of adding extra oils beyond what is needed for saponification. A common superfat percentage is around 5%, which helps ensure your soap is moisturizing and not drying. You can adjust the superfat percentage in SoapCalc to see how it affects the lye calculation.

- Curing Times: While the calculator does not directly provide curing times, it's essential to remember that goat milk soaps typically require 4-6 weeks to cure. This allows the soap to harden and the lye to fully saponify, ensuring a safe and gentle product.

By utilizing SoapCalc effectively, you can create customized goat milk soap recipes that cater to your specific needs and preferences. This tool empowers you to experiment confidently, ensuring that each batch of soap is both safe and enjoyable to use. Happy soap-making!

Section 5: Tailoring Soap for Specific Skin Needs

1. Sensitive Skin: Calming Calendula Soap

Recipe Tailored for Sensitive and Inflamed Skin:

Ingredients:

- 16 oz. (1 lb.) goat milk (frozen)

- 6 oz. lye (sodium hydroxide)

- 32 oz. (2 lb.) olive oil

- 16 oz. (1 lb.) coconut oil

- 16 oz. (1 lb.) almond oil

- 2 tablespoons dried calendula petals

- 4 oz. calendula-infused oil (made by infusing olive oil with calendula flowers)

- Optional: 1 oz chamomile essential oil for added soothing properties

Step-by-Step Instructions:

1. Prepare Your Workspace: Ensure your workspace is clean and well-ventilated. Gather all the necessary tools and ingredients.

2. Infuse the Oil: To make calendula-infused oil, combine dried calendula petals with olive oil in a jar and let it sit in a warm, sunny spot for 1-2 weeks, shaking it occasionally. Strain the oil before use.

3. Freeze the Goat Milk: Freeze the goat milk in ice cube trays until solid.

4. Mix the Lye Solution: In a well-ventilated area, carefully measure the lye. Slowly add the lye to the frozen goat milk while stirring gently. Allow it to cool to around 100-110°F (38-43°C).

5. Melt the Oils: In a separate pot, combine the coconut oil, almond oil, and calendula-infused olive oil. Heat gently until melted and combined. Allow to cool to about 100-110°F (38-43°C).

6. Combine Lye and Oils: Once both the lye solution and oils are at the same temperature, slowly pour the lye solution into the oils while blending with a stick blender until you reach trace.

7. Add Dried Calendula and Optional Essential Oil: At trace, add the dried calendula petals and chamomile essential oil, mixing thoroughly.

8. Pour into Mold: Carefully pour the soap mixture into your mold, smoothing the top with a spatula.

9. Cure the Soap: Cover the mold with a towel and allow it to sit for 24-48 hours until hardened. Remove from the mold and cut into bars.

10. Cure the Bars: Place the bars on a drying rack in a cool, dry area for 4-6 weeks to cure.

Discussion on the Soothing Properties of Calendula

Calendula is renowned for its soothing and anti-inflammatory properties, making it an excellent choice for sensitive and inflamed skin. It can help reduce redness and irritation, promoting healing and comfort. The natural compounds in calendula have been shown to support skin regeneration, making this soap particularly beneficial for those with conditions like eczema or dermatitis. Additionally, its gentle nature makes it suitable for all skin types, including babies and those with very sensitive skin.

2. Oily Skin: Lemon and Charcoal Soap

Recipe Focused on Oil Control and Detoxification:

Ingredients:

- 16 oz. (1 lb.) goat milk (frozen)

- 6 oz. lye (sodium hydroxide)

- 32 oz. (2 lb.) olive oil

- 16 oz. (1 lb.) coconut oil

- 16 oz. (1 lb.) almond oil

- 2 tablespoons activated charcoal

- 1 oz. lemon essential oil

Optional: Zest of one lemon for added texture and fragrance

Instructions for Incorporating Coffee Grounds and Sea Salt:

1. Prepare Your Workspace: Ensure your workspace is clean and well-ventilated. Gather all the necessary tools and ingredients.

2. Freeze the Goat Milk: Freeze the goat milk in ice cube trays until solid.

3. Mix the Lye Solution: In a well-ventilated area, carefully measure the lye. Slowly add the lye to the frozen goat milk while stirring gently. Allow it to cool to around 100-110°F (38-43°C).

4. Melt the Oils: In a separate pot, combine the coconut oil, almond oil, and olive oil. Heat gently until melted and combined. Allow to cool to about 100-110°F (38-43°C).

5. Combine Lye and Oils: Once both the lye solution and oils are at the same temperature, slowly pour the lye solution into the oils while blending with a stick blender until you reach trace.

6. Add Activated Charcoal and Essential Oil: At trace, add the activated charcoal and lemon essential oil. If using, add the lemon zest for additional texture and fragrance. Mix thoroughly to ensure even distribution.

7. Pour into Mold: Carefully pour the soap mixture into your mold, smoothing the top with a spatula.

8. Cure the Soap: Cover the mold with a towel and allow it to sit for 24-48 hours until hardened. Remove from the mold and cut into bars.

9. Cure the Bars: Place the bars on a drying rack in a cool, dry area for 4-6 weeks to cure.

Benefits of Using Activated Charcoal and Lemon Zest

Activated charcoal is a powerful natural detoxifier that helps draw out impurities and excess oil from the skin. It can effectively unclog pores, making it an excellent choice for those with oily or acne-prone skin. The addition of lemon zest and lemon essential oil not only provides a refreshing citrus scent but also offers astringent properties that can help tighten pores and control oil production. Together, these ingredients create a soap that cleanses deeply while leaving the skin feeling fresh and revitalized.

By tailoring your soap recipes to address specific skin needs, you can create effective and nourishing products that enhance your skincare routine. Enjoy the process of crafting these specialized soaps and the benefits they bring to your skin!

Section 6: The Role of Additives in Soap Making

Explanation of Various Additives

Additives play a crucial role in soap making, enhancing both the functional and aesthetic qualities of the final product. Here are some common additives and their benefits:

- Honey: Known for its moisturizing and antibacterial properties, honey can help hydrate the skin and promote healing. It also adds a natural sweetness and a lovely golden hue to the soap.

- Oatmeal: A gentle exfoliant, oatmeal is excellent for soothing irritated skin. It can help relieve dryness and is particularly beneficial for sensitive skin types. Ground oatmeal can also add texture to the soap.

- Clays: Natural clays, such as bentonite or kaolin, can be used to absorb excess oil and impurities from the skin. They also provide a smooth texture and can enhance the soap's color.

- Aloe Vera: Renowned for its soothing and hydrating properties, aloe vera can help calm inflamed skin and provide moisture. It is often used in soaps aimed at sensitive or sunburned skin.

These additives not only improve the skin benefits of the soap but also contribute to its appearance and texture.

Methods for Incorporating Additives Without Altering Soap Texture

Incorporating additives into your soap without compromising its texture requires careful consideration. Here are some effective methods:

1. Timing of Addition: Additives should be incorporated at the right stage of the soap-making process. For instance, honey and aloe vera can be added at trace, while clays and oatmeal can be mixed into the oils before combining with the lye solution.

2. Proper Measurements: Use recommended usage rates for each additive to avoid altering the soap's consistency. For example, adding too much honey can cause the soap to become overly soft, while excessive clay can make it too thick.

3. Pre-Mixing: For powdered additives like clays and oatmeal, pre-mixing them with a small amount of oil before adding them to the soap can help prevent clumping and ensure even distribution.

4. Infusions: Infusing oils with herbs or botanicals (like calendula or chamomile) before soap making can enhance the properties of the soap without altering its texture. This method allows for a more uniform incorporation of the beneficial properties.

Tips for Experimenting with New Additives

Experimenting with new additives can be a fun and rewarding part of soap making. Here are some tips to help you get started:

- Start Small: When trying a new additive, begin with a small batch to test its effects on the soap's texture and performance. This allows you to make adjustments without wasting materials.

- Research Properties: Understand the properties of the additives you want to use. Some may require specific handling or have particular effects on the saponification process.

- Document Your Process: Keep detailed notes on the amounts and types of additives used and the results. This will help you replicate successful batches or adjust future recipes based on your findings.

- Combine Additives: Don't hesitate to mix different additives to create unique blends. For example, combining honey with oatmeal can enhance both moisturizing and exfoliating properties.

- Seek Feedback: Share your creations with friends or family to gather feedback on texture, scent, and skin feel. This can provide valuable insights for future batches.

By understanding the role of additives and how to incorporate them effectively, you can enhance your soap-making skills and create products that cater to specific skin needs while also being aesthetically pleasing. Enjoy the creative process of experimenting with different additives to find the perfect combinations for your soap!

Section 7: Personal Favorites and Inspirations

In the world of soap making, each recipe has a story—a blend of experiences and inspirations that shape our creative journey. Here are some of my personal favorite soap recipes, each accompanied by its unique backstory and the creative process behind it.

Favorite Recipe 1: Lavender and Honey Oatmeal Soap

o Backstory: This soap was inspired by a peaceful day in my garden surrounded by blooming lavender and buzzing bees. The serene environment encouraged me to focus on self-care and mindfulness.

Inspiration and Creative Process:

I combined high-quality lavender essential oils, honey from my favorite local beekeepers, and colloidal gluten-free oatmeal to create a soap that promotes relaxation and healing. This soap serves as a gentle reminder to take time for oneself, making it a delightful gift for friends seeking tranquility.

Favorite Recipe 2: Coffee & Vanilla

o   Backstory: This recipe is a sweet vision of mornings with my husband: hot cups of coffee in our hands, with the scent of vanilla in the air, enjoying each other's company.

Inspiration and Creative Process:

To capture those nostalgic mornings, I used our favorite coffee grinds blended with the best vanilla I have ever tasted to create a luxurious and mildly exfoliating soap.

Favorite Recipe 3: Pumpkin Cinnamon Swirl

o   Backstory: Inspired by afternoons spent in my pumpkin patch, spices in the air when baking in the kitchen, and the cool fall air signaling the changes of the season.

Inspiration and Creative Process:

I used pumpkin puree from my garden, a beautiful blend of spices like cinnamon, ginger, nutmeg, allspice, cloves, and essential oils. This soap not only cleanses but also offers a nurturing touch to the skin and reminds me of the most delicious pumpkin pie piping hot from the oven,

Section 8: Encouraging Experimentation and Creativity

Soap making is an art that thrives on experimentation and creativity. Here are some tips and encouragement for soap makers looking to explore new ingredients and techniques.

Tips on Documenting and Tweaking Recipes

- Keep a Detailed Record: Maintain a soap-making journal where you document each recipe, including ingredients, measurements, and the process. Note any variations or adjustments made during the soap-making process for future reference.

- Track Results: After each batch, record observations about texture, scent, and skin feel. This information will help you refine your recipes and understand how different ingredients interact.

- Experiment Gradually: When trying new ingredients or techniques, start with small batches. This allows you to tweak and adjust without wasting materials while developing your skills.

Encouragement to Explore New Ingredients and Techniques

- Be Bold: Don't shy away from experimenting with unique additives like exotic oils, herbs, and natural colorants. Each new ingredient can bring a fresh perspective and enhance the properties of your soap.

- Learn from Others: Join soap-making communities or forums where you can share ideas and gain inspiration from fellow soap makers. Engaging with others can spark creativity and introduce you to new techniques.

Advice on Maintaining a Soap-Making Journal and Sharing Discoveries

- Create a Dedicated Journal: Use a notebook or digital platform to organize your soap-making journey. Include sections for recipes, ingredient notes, and personal reflections on each batch.

- Share Your Discoveries: Whether through social media, blogs, or local workshops, sharing your experiences can inspire others and foster a sense of community. Highlight your successes and even your failures, as both can offer valuable lessons.

By documenting your soap-making journey and encouraging creativity, you can develop your skills and discover new possibilities. Embrace the art of experimentation and let your imagination guide you in crafting unique and beautiful soaps!

The journey of soap making is a truly rewarding experience that combines creativity, science, and personal expression. Each bar of custom soap is not just a cleansing product; it embodies the love and care put into its creation. From selecting the finest ingredients to experimenting with unique fragrances and textures, the process allows for endless possibilities and personal storytelling.

Creating custom soaps offers a sense of accomplishment that is hard to match. The satisfaction of crafting something beautiful and beneficial for yourself or others is a joy that resonates deeply. Each successful batch brings a sense of pride, while even the occasional mishap serves as a valuable learning opportunity, adding to the richness of your soap-making journey.

As you explore the world of soap making, I encourage you to keep pushing the boundaries of your creativity. Experiment with new ingredients, techniques, and combinations. Don't be afraid to take risks and try something outside your comfort zone—this is where the magic happens! Document your findings, refine your recipes, and allow your unique style to shine through.

Remember, the beauty of soap making lies not only in the finished product but in the process itself. Enjoy every moment of your craft, share your discoveries with others, and let your passion for soap making flourish. The joy of creating custom soaps is a journey worth embracing, and I hope it continues to inspire you for years to come!

Appendix: Additional Resources

For those eager to expand their soap-making knowledge, here's a concise list of valuable resources, including books, websites, communities, and suppliers.

1. Recommended Books

   o *"The Complete Soapmaker," by Anne L. Watson*

A thorough guide covering basic techniques to advanced recipes, ideal for all skill levels.

   o *"Soap Crafting: Step-by-Step Techniques for Making 31 Unique Cold Process Soaps," by Anne-Marie Faiola*

Offers detailed instructions and creative ideas for crafting stunning cold process soaps.

o *"The Natural Soap Book," by Susan Millerick*

Focuses on eco-friendly recipes and techniques using natural ingredients.

2. Websites

o *Soap Queen*

Features over 100 videos on soap-making techniques, lye safety, and ingredient usage.

o *The Nova Studio*

Provides free resources, including videos and worksheets, perfect for beginners.

o *Countryside*

Simplifies the soap-making process with clear instructions for various soap types.

3. Online Communities

o *Facebook Groups*

Join groups like "Lovin Soap Project" to connect, share ideas, and seek advice from fellow soap makers.

o *Reddit*

Engage with the vibrant r/soapmaking subreddit to ask questions and share your creations.

Suppliers for Soap-Making Supplies and Ingredients

o *Windy Point Soapmaking Supplies*

My favorite Canadian supply store for oils, powders, some packaging and additives.

o *Bramble Berry*

A reliable source for soap-making ingredients, offering tutorials and recipes.

o *Wholesale Supplies Plus*

Provides an extensive range of supplies and resources for all skill levels.

o *Mountain Rose Herbs*

Specializes in natural ingredients, offering high-quality herbs and essential oils.

By leveraging these resources, you can enhance your soap-making skills, connect with a community of enthusiasts, and explore the vast creative possibilities of this craft. Happy soap making!

∽○

Chapter Eight:
Other Things to Make with Goat Milk Soap

Goat milk is a versatile ingredient that extends far beyond traditional soap. While goat milk soap may be the first product that comes to mind, this rich and nourishing ingredient can be used to craft a wide range of luxurious bath and body care items.

In this chapter, we will explore the various ways you can harness the benefits of goat milk to create products that complement and go beyond traditional soap. From soothing bath bombs to hydrating lotion bars, we will delve into recipes, techniques, and customization tips to help you make high-quality, artisanal products that elevate everyday self-care.

Whether you're crafting for personal use, creating thoughtful gifts, or developing a product line for sale, the possibilities with goat milk are endless.

Get ready to unlock the full potential of this versatile ingredient and discover new ways to pamper your skin with luxurious, natural bath and body care products.

The Versatility of Goat Milk Beyond Soap

Goat milk is renowned for its exceptional nourishing properties, making it a prized ingredient in skincare. Rich in vitamins A, D, and E, as well as essential fatty acids and minerals, goat milk provides deep hydration and supports healthy skin.

Its natural lactic acid gently exfoliates, promoting smoother, more radiant skin, while its anti-inflammatory properties help soothe conditions such as eczema, psoriasis, and dryness.

While goat milk soap is a popular choice for gentle cleansing, the benefits of goat milk extend far beyond. Its creamy, moisturizing nature makes it an ideal base for a variety of bath and body care products, including lotions, bath bombs, lip balms, and salves.

These products harness the same nourishing qualities as soap, offering a complete skincare routine that leaves the skin feeling soft, hydrated, and refreshed.

For individuals with sensitive skin, goat milk-based products provide a natural, chemical-free alternative to synthetic skincare. Unlike many commercial products that contain harsh chemicals, goat milk is gentle and non-irritating, making it suitable for all skin types.

Bath Bombs: Effervescent Luxury

Bath bombs have become a staple of self-care routines, transforming an ordinary bath into a spa-like experience with their effervescent fizz and delightful scents. When infused with goat milk, bath bombs take on an added layer of luxury, offering both relaxation and skin-nourishing benefits.

Benefits of Goat Milk in Bath Bombs

- Hydration and Skin Nourishment: Goat milk is rich in essential fatty acids and vitamins, making it a powerful moisturizer. When added to bath bombs, it helps to hydrate and soften the skin, leaving it feeling smooth and supple. The lactic acid in goat milk also gently exfoliates, promoting a healthier, more radiant complexion.

- Soothing Properties: Bath bombs with goat milk are especially beneficial for individuals with dry or irritated skin. Goat milk's anti-inflammatory properties help calm redness, itching, and irritation, making it an excellent choice for those with sensitive skin or conditions like eczema and psoriasis. Combined with the relaxing experience of a warm bath, these bath bombs provide both physical and emotional relief.

Basic Goat Milk Bath Bomb Recipe

Ingredients:

- 1 cup baking soda

- 1/2 cup citric acid

- 1/2 cup cornstarch

- 1/4 cup goat milk powder

- 2 tablespoons carrier oil (such as coconut, almond, or jojoba)

- 1 teaspoon water or witch hazel (adjust as needed)

- 10–15 drops of essential oils (lavender, eucalyptus, or citrus)

- Natural colorants (optional)

- Silicone or plastic molds

Crafting Luxurious Goat Milk Bath Bombs

1. Mix the Dry Ingredients: In a large bowl, combine the baking soda, citric acid, cornstarch, and goat milk powder. Whisk thoroughly to remove any clumps and ensure even distribution.

2. Add the Wet Ingredients: In a separate bowl, mix the carrier oil, essential oils, and a small amount of water or witch hazel. Slowly add the wet mixture to the dry ingredients, stirring continuously. Be careful not to add too much liquid at once, as it can cause the mixture to fizz prematurely.

3. Adjust the Texture: The mixture should have a consistency similar to damp sand. If it's too dry, add a few more drops of water or witch hazel. If it's too wet, add a little more baking soda.

4. Molding: Quickly pack the mixture into the molds, pressing firmly to ensure the bath bombs hold their shape. Smooth the surface and gently tap the molds to release the bath bombs onto a flat surface.

5. Drying: Allow the bath bombs to air dry for 24–48 hours in a cool, dry place. Once fully hardened, they're ready to use or package as gifts.

Customization Ideas for Luxurious Goat Milk Bath Bombs

- Flower Petals or Herbs: Incorporate dried lavender, rose petals, or chamomile into the mixture for a natural, decorative touch.

- Glitter: For a fun, sparkling effect, add a pinch of biodegradable glitter.

- Color Variations: Use natural colorants like beetroot powder, spirulina, or turmeric to create beautiful, vibrant bath bombs without synthetic dyes.

- Scent Combinations: Experiment with different essential oil blends to create unique scents. For a calming experience, try lavender and chamomile. For an energizing bath, opt for citrus and mint.

With these customization ideas, you can turn a simple bath into a luxurious escape, providing both relaxation and skincare in one delightful product. The addition of goat milk offers hydration and soothing properties, making these bath bombs a truly indulgent experience.

Bath Salts: Therapeutic Relaxation

Bath salts have long been used to enhance the bathing experience, offering therapeutic benefits that soothe both the body and mind. When enriched with goat milk, bath salts provide an added layer of nourishment, transforming a simple soak into a luxurious, spa-like treatment.

Benefits of Goat Milk Bath Salts

- Relieves Muscle Tension The combination of Epsom salt and sea salt in bath salts helps to ease muscle soreness and tension. Magnesium, a key component of Epsom salt, is absorbed through the skin, promoting relaxation and relieving fatigue. When paired with goat milk, the bath becomes a rejuvenating experience that soothes both muscles and skin.

- Exfoliates and Softens Skin Goat milk powder in bath salts gently exfoliates, removing dead skin cells and revealing smoother, softer skin. The lactic acid in goat milk helps to brighten the skin, while its vitamins and minerals provide deep hydration, making it an excellent choice for individuals with dry or sensitive skin.

Recipe for Goat Milk Bath Salts

Ingredients:

- 1 cup Epsom salt

- 1/2 cup sea salt (fine or coarse)

- 1/4 cup goat milk powder

- 10–15 drops of essential oils (lavender, eucalyptus, or your preferred scent)

- 2 tablespoons dried herbs (such as lavender buds, rose petals, or chamomile)

- Natural colorants (optional)

Crafting Luxurious Goat Milk Bath Salts

1. Mix the Salts: In a large bowl, combine the Epsom salt and sea salt. Mix well to ensure an even distribution.

2. Add Goat Milk Powder: Gently stir in the goat milk powder, making sure it is evenly incorporated into the salt mixture.

3. Incorporate Essential Oils: Add your chosen essential oils, a few drops at a time, and mix thoroughly. Adjust the amount based on the desired strength of the fragrance.

4. Add Dried Herbs and Colorants: If using dried herbs or natural colorants, fold them into the mixture. Herbs like lavender, chamomile, or rose petals not only add visual appeal but also enhance the therapeutic properties of the bath salts.

5. Layer or Mix: For a visually appealing product, you can layer the salts, goat milk powder, and herbs in a glass jar, creating distinct layers of each ingredient. Alternatively, mix everything together for a uniform appearance.

6. Store and Use: Transfer the bath salts to an airtight container. To use, simply add 1/4 to 1/2 cup of the mixture to warm bathwater, allowing it to dissolve fully before soaking.

Tips for Creating Aromatherapy Blends for Goat Milk Bath Salts

- Relaxation Blend Essential Oils: Lavender, chamomile, and ylang-ylang Herbs: Lavender buds or dried chamomile flowers Benefits: Promotes relaxation, reduces stress, and improves sleep quality.

- Refreshing Blend Essential Oils: Eucalyptus, peppermint, and lemon Herbs: Dried mint leaves or lemon peel Benefits: Energizes the body, clears the mind, and soothes tired muscles.

- Skin-Soothing Blend Essential Oils: Rose, geranium, and frankincense Herbs: Dried rose petals and calendula Benefits: Hydrates and nourishes the skin while providing anti-inflammatory properties.

Goat Milk Lotion Bars: Solid Skin Nourishment

Lotion bars are a convenient and effective way to keep skin moisturized, providing all the benefits of a traditional lotion in a solid, easy-to-use form. When enriched with goat milk, these bars deliver deep hydration and skin nourishment, making them a versatile addition to any skincare routine.

Goat milk, with its natural emollient properties, helps to soften and smooth the skin. The lactic acid in goat milk gently exfoliates, while the vitamins and minerals nourish and replenish the skin. By incorporating goat milk into lotion bars, you can create a luxurious, moisturizing experience that leaves the skin feeling soft, supple, and healthy.

These solid lotion bars are easy to use and travel-friendly, making them a convenient option for on-the-go hydration. Simply rub the bar onto clean, dry skin, and the warmth of your body will melt the bar, allowing the nourishing ingredients to be absorbed. The solid format also helps to minimize waste, as you can control the amount of product used with each application.

Whether you're looking to soothe dry, cracked skin, nourish delicate areas, or maintain overall skin health, goat milk lotion bars offer a versatile and effective solution. Incorporate them into your daily skincare routine for a luxurious and hydrating experience.

Advantages of Goat Milk Lotion Bars

- Portable and Spill-Proof Unlike traditional liquid lotions, lotion bars are solid and compact, making them perfect for travel or keeping in a purse or pocket. There's no risk of spills or leaks, and they can be used on the go for quick hydration.

- Long-Lasting Moisturization Lotion bars are formulated with rich butters, oils, and waxes that create a protective barrier on the skin, locking in moisture for hours. Goat milk's natural emollients enhance this effect, leaving the skin soft, smooth, and nourished.

Recipe for Goat Milk Lotion Bars

Ingredients:

- 1/4 cup beeswax (grated or pellets)

- 1/4 cup shea butter (or cocoa butter)

- 1/4 cup carrier oil (such as coconut oil, almond oil, or jojoba oil)

- 1 tablespoon goat milk powder

- 10–15 drops of essential oils (optional, for fragrance)

- Silicone deodorant tubes or metal tins for shaping

Instructions:

1. Melt the Ingredients: In a double boiler, combine the beeswax, shea butter, and carrier oil. Heat gently, stirring occasionally, until all ingredients are fully melted and combined.

2. Add Goat Milk Powder: Once the mixture is melted, remove it from the heat and allow it to cool slightly. Stir in the goat milk powder, ensuring it is fully dissolved and evenly distributed.

3. Add Essential Oils: If desired, add 10–15 drops of essential oils to the mixture. Stir well to incorporate. Popular choices include lavender for relaxation, citrus for a refreshing scent, or vanilla for a warm, comforting fragrance.

4. Pour into deodorant tubes: Carefully pour the mixture into silicone deodorant tubes or metal tins. Allow the lotion bars to cool and harden completely at room temperature, which may take several hours.

5. Remove and Store: Once fully hardened, gently pop the lotion bars out of the deodorant tubes. Store them in a cool, dry place or package them in tins or reusable containers for personal use or gifting.

Seasonal Variations for Handmade Soap

Summer Citrus Bars

- Essential Oils: Lemon, lime, and grapefruit

- Additions: A small amount of mica powder for a subtle shimmer

- Benefits: Provides a refreshing, uplifting scent and light hydration ideal for warmer months.

Winter Warmth Bars

- Essential Oils: Vanilla, cinnamon, and clove

- Additions: A pinch of ground cinnamon for a warm, festive touch

- Benefits: Deeply hydrates dry winter skin while offering a comforting, cozy scent.

Floral Spring Bars

- Essential Oils: Rose, lavender, and geranium

- Additions: Dried flower petals for a decorative finish

- Benefits: Softens and nourishes the skin while imparting a delicate floral fragrance.

Goat milk lotion bars are a luxurious and practical way to keep skin moisturized year-round. With endless customization options, they can be tailored to fit any season or personal preference, making them a perfect addition to any skincare collection or a thoughtful handmade gift.

Lip Balms and Salves: Lip and Skin Care Essentials

Lips and skin require extra care, especially during harsh weather conditions. With its nourishing and hydrating properties, goat milk is an excellent ingredient for lip balms and salves, offering soothing relief and long-lasting moisture.

Benefits of Goat Milk for Lips and Skin

- Hydrates and Repairs Chapped Lips

Goat milk is rich in fatty acids, vitamins, and minerals that provide deep hydration, making it ideal for restoring moisture to dry, cracked lips. Its natural emollients soften the lips while its lactic acid gently exfoliates, leaving them smooth and supple.

- Soothes and Heals Dry Skin

When used in salves, goat milk helps to calm irritated skin, reduce inflammation, and promote healing of minor cuts, burns, and dry patches. Its nourishing properties make it a versatile addition to skincare products designed for targeted relief.

Recipe for Goat Milk Lip Balm

Ingredients:

- 1 tablespoon beeswax (grated or pellets)

- 1 tablespoon coconut oil

- 1 tablespoon shea butter (or cocoa butter)

- 1 teaspoon goat milk powder

- 5–10 drops natural flavoring oils (such as vanilla, peppermint, or citrus)

- Optional: Natural colorants (beetroot powder or mica) for a tinted balm

- Lip balm tubes or tins

Instructions:

Here are the steps to make your own homemade lip balm:

1. Melt the Base Ingredients: In a double boiler, melt the beeswax, coconut oil, and shea butter over low heat. Stir until fully melted and combined.

2. Add Goat Milk Powder: Remove the mixture from heat and allow it to cool slightly. Stir in the goat milk powder, ensuring it dissolves completely.

3. Incorporate Flavoring Oils: Add 5–10 drops of your chosen flavoring oil and stir well. For a tinted balm, mix in a small amount of natural colorant until the desired shade is achieved.

4. Pour into Containers: Carefully pour the mixture into lip balm tubes or tins. Allow the balms to cool and harden completely before sealing the containers.

5. Store and Use: Store the lip balms in a cool, dry place. Apply as needed to hydrate and protect your lips.

Customization Ideas for Homemade Lip Balm

Tinted Balm

To create a tinted lip balm, add beetroot powder for a soft pink hue or mica for a subtle shimmer.

Healing Balm

To create a healing lip balm, add a few drops of vitamin E oil for additional healing and antioxidant properties.

Recipe for Healing Salves

Ingredients:

- 1/4 cup infused herbal oil (such as calendula, chamomile, or lavender)

- 1 tablespoon beeswax

- 1 tablespoon shea butter or cocoa butter

- 1 teaspoon goat milk powder

- 10–15 drops essential oils (tea tree for antiseptic properties, lavender for soothing, or frankincense for healing)

- Small tins or glass jars

Instructions:

1. Prepare the Herbal Oil: If you don't have infused herbal oil, prepare it by steeping dried herbs in a carrier oil (such as olive or almond oil) for 1–2 weeks. Strain the oil before use.

2. Melt the Beeswax and Butter: In a double boiler, melt the beeswax and shea butter together. Once melted, add the infused herbal oil and stir until well combined.

3. Add Goat Milk Powder: Remove from heat and stir in the goat milk powder until fully incorporated.

4. Incorporate Essential Oils: Add 10–15 drops of your chosen essential oils and mix thoroughly.

5. Pour into Containers: Carefully pour the salve mixture into small tins or glass jars. Allow it to cool and solidify completely.

6. Store and Use: Store the salve in a cool, dry place. Use it on minor cuts, burns, dry patches, or other areas needing extra care.

Creating Themed Gift Sets: A Thoughtful Touch for Every Occasion

Handmade goat milk products offer the perfect foundation for creating luxurious, personalized gift sets. Whether for holidays, birthdays, or special occasions, themed sets can transform your creations into memorable gifts that delight the senses and provide a unique, spa-like experience.

Designing Coordinated Gift Sets

When crafting gift sets, a cohesive theme ties the products together and enhances their overall appeal. Here are some creative ideas for themed gift sets:

1. Relaxation Set

Designed for those in need of stress relief and self-care, this set features calming scents and soothing products.

Contents:

- Lavender-scented goat milk bath bombs for a calming, fizzy soak.

- Lavender-infused goat milk bath salts to relax muscles and soften skin.

- Moisturizing lavender-scented goat milk lotion bars for post-bath hydration.

Additional Touch: Include a lavender sachet or a small soy candle for a complete relaxation experience.

2. Winter Care Kit

Perfect for combating dry, winter skin, this kit offers rich, nourishing products to keep skin soft and hydrated during the colder months.

Contents:

- Vanilla-scented goat milk lotion bars for deep hydration.

- Peppermint-flavored lip balm to soothe and protect chapped lips.

- A bar of creamy goat milk soap with a wintery, festive scent like cinnamon or pine.

Additional Touch: Add a pair of cozy socks or a sachet of herbal tea to enhance the winter comfort theme.

3. Spa Day Package

Bring the luxury of a spa into the home with this indulgent set of pampering products.

Contents:

- Rose-scented goat milk bath salts for a rejuvenating soak.

- A rose-infused sugar scrub to gently exfoliate and reveal smooth, glowing skin.

- A coordinating goat milk soap with a matching floral fragrance.

Additional Touch: Include a loofah, a facial mask, or a small bottle of essential oil to elevate the spa experience.

Packaging Tips

Beautiful and thoughtful packaging elevates the value of your gift sets and leaves a lasting impression. Consider these tips for eco-friendly and aesthetically pleasing presentation:

Eco-Friendly Packaging Options

- Kraft Paper Boxes: These biodegradable boxes provide a rustic, natural look and are perfect for a minimalist aesthetic.

- Glass Jars: Ideal for bath salts and scrubs, glass jars can be reused by the recipient, adding an eco-conscious touch to your gift.

- Fabric Wraps: Use reusable fabric wraps, such as muslin or patterned cotton, for a zero-waste packaging option that looks elegant and unique.

Adding Personalized Touches

- Handwritten Notes: Include a personalized note expressing well wishes or describing the products in the set. This small gesture adds a heartfelt touch.

- Ribbon Ties: Use ribbons, twine, or raffia to secure the packaging and add a decorative element that complements the theme of the set.

- Custom Tags: Create custom labels or tags that reflect the theme of the gift set. Include details about the products, such as ingredients or suggested use, to add a professional touch.

Experimenting with Scents, Textures, and Additives: Crafting Unique Goat Milk Products

One of the greatest advantages of working with goat milk is the ability to customize each product with a variety of scents, textures, and skin-nourishing additives. By experimenting with different combinations, you can create a range of unique products that cater to various skin types, preferences, and needs.

Scent Combinations: Crafting the Perfect Fragrance Profiles

Scent plays a major role in the sensory experience of bath products, evoking emotions and enhancing relaxation. With goat milk's mild, creamy base, it pairs beautifully with a range of essential oils to create signature scents. Here are some combinations to consider:

Scent Combinations: Crafting the Perfect Fragrance Profiles

1. Floral: Lavender + Rose

   - Fragrance Profile: Soft, calming, and romantic.

- Uses: Lavender's soothing properties combine with the floral sweetness of rose to create a gentle, relaxing scent perfect for bedtime routines or stress relief.

2. Herbal: Eucalyptus + Mint

   - Fragrance Profile: Invigorating, refreshing, and cool.

   - Uses: Eucalyptus and mint are great for clearing sinuses and refreshing the senses, making this combination ideal for an uplifting, energizing bath or a wake-me-up shower.

3. Citrus: Orange + Lemon

   - Fragrance Profile: Bright, fresh, and energizing.

   - Uses: Perfect for a morning pick-me-up, this combination stimulates the senses and adds a burst of freshness to your skincare products, especially in summer.

4. Sweet: Vanilla + Almond

   - Fragrance Profile: Warm, cozy, and sweet.

   - Uses: Vanilla is rich and comforting, while almond offers a nutty, subtle sweetness, making this scent combination ideal for body butters and lotion bars designed for dry skin.

Texture Variations: Customizing Feel and Function

Different textures enhance the experience of using your goat milk products, whether you're looking for something that exfoliates, moisturizes, or nourishes. Here are some ways to experiment with textures:

Texture Variations: Customizing Feel and Function

1. Exfoliating: Adding texture for a gentle scrub

    *   Exfoliants: Sugar, oatmeal, or coffee grounds.

    *   Effect: These natural exfoliants help slough off dead skin cells, leaving the skin smooth and refreshed. Ideal for scrubs or bath bombs, exfoliating ingredients provide a deep-cleaning experience while offering additional skin benefits like increased circulation.

Tip: Oatmeal is especially great for sensitive skin, as it soothes and calms irritation while gently exfoliating.

2. Creamy: Increasing hydration and smoothness

    *   Ingredients: Butters like shea butter, cocoa butter, or mango butter; oils like coconut, almond, or jojoba.

    *   Effect: A higher ratio of rich butters and oils will yield a creamy, moisturizing product that's perfect for dry or dehydrated skin. These ingredients give products a luxurious feel and help lock in moisture for hours.

Tip: Use creamy variations for products like lotion bars, lip balms, and body butters, where long-lasting hydration is key.

Additives for Skin Benefits: Targeting Specific Needs

Adding natural, skin-friendly ingredients to your goat milk products allows you to tailor your creations to address various skincare concerns. Here are a few powerful additives to experiment with:

1. Dried Herbs: Chamomile and Calendula

   - Chamomile: Known for its anti-inflammatory properties, chamomile calms irritated skin and reduces redness. It's perfect for sensitive skin or anyone seeking soothing relief after sun exposure or harsh weather.

   - Calendula: Often used for its skin-healing abilities, calendula helps with cuts, bruises, and other minor skin irritations. It's great for those with dry or inflamed skin.

2. Clays: Kaolin and Bentonite

   - Kaolin Clay: A gentle clay perfect for sensitive skin. It absorbs excess oil and impurities without over-drying or irritating. Ideal for creating gentle face masks or soaps for delicate skin.

   - Bentonite Clay: Known for its ability to detoxify and draw out impurities, bentonite clay is excellent for oily or acne-prone skin. Use it in face masks or soaps designed to balance and clarify the skin.

Labeling and Packaging for Sales or Gifts: Presenting Your Goat Milk Products with Care

When creating goat milk products for sale or as gifts, the packaging and labeling are just as important as the quality of the products themselves. Thoughtful and effective labeling not only informs consumers but also enhances the overall aesthetic of the product, helping it stand out in the crowded marketplace. Whether you're looking to build a brand or gift a personalized set, here are some tips to make your goat milk products shine with proper labeling and packaging:

The Importance of Proper Labeling

Proper labeling is essential for ensuring that your products are safe, transparent, and user-friendly. It builds trust with your customers, particularly when they are using skincare products.

Here are some key elements to include on your product labels:

Ingredients

- Why it's important: Listing the ingredients in your products shows transparency and helps consumers make informed choices, especially those with allergies or sensitivities. For example, if your bath bombs contain coconut oil, it's crucial to list it so individuals with coconut allergies can avoid it.

- What to include: A full ingredient list that uses the common names of ingredients. For example, "Cocos Nucifera Oil" (coconut oil) or "Butyrospermum Parkii" (shea butter). Be sure to mention any essential oils, natural fragrances, and colorants.

Tip: If you use any preservatives, be sure to note those too, especially if they are synthetic or have a potential for irritation.

Usage Instructions and Storage Tips

- Why it's important: Customers need to know how to use the product to get the best results. Providing clear instructions ensures that your customers have the best possible experience and don't end up misusing the product.

- What to include: Detailed usage instructions—whether to apply the lotion bar after a bath or how much bath salt to use in a full tub of water.

Storage Tips: Since goat milk-based products may require specific care (e.g., refrigeration for lotions or keeping out of direct sunlight), include helpful storage tips. This can prolong the shelf life of the product and prevent it from degrading.

Expiration Date to Ensure Product Safety

- Why it's important: Natural products like goat milk soaps and lotions may not have a long shelf life, and it's important to indicate when a product should be used by to ensure it's still effective and safe.

- What to include: A clear expiration date or a "Best Used By" date based on when the product was made. If you make small batches, it's easy to track this. Additionally, if you sell in larger quantities, consider indicating a timeframe for optimal use (e.g., within 6 months of purchase).

Designing Eye-Catching Labels

Crafting an effective product label is crucial for attracting customers and reflecting your brand's identity. Here are some key tips for designing eye-catching labels:

1. Use Fonts, Colors, and Graphics that Align with the Product's Theme: The visual elements of your label should complement the essence of the product. Choose fonts, colors, and graphics that evoke the mood and benefits of the item.

- Fonts: Select fonts that are easy to read but also reflect the feel of your brand. For example, script fonts may work well for luxurious, spa-like products, while clean sans-serif fonts are great for minimalist designs.

- Colors: Soft pastel shades can work well for gentle, soothing products, while bold, bright colors can convey freshness and energy. Use a consistent color palette that matches your brand identity.

- Graphics: Incorporate relevant imagery that reflects the natural ingredients and the product's benefits, such as floral designs for lavender-scented products or clean, minimal graphics for eco-friendly lines.

2. Incorporate Brand Logos and Contact Information for Marketing Purposes: Prominently displaying your brand logo and including clear contact information makes your product easily identifiable and provides customers with a way to learn more about your brand.

- Logo: Ensure your logo is prominent on the label, so your brand is immediately recognizable.

- Contact Information: Include your business's website, email address, and social media handles, if applicable. This allows customers to learn more about your products, make repeat purchases, or share their experiences on social media.

- Tagline or Message: A catchy tagline that captures the essence of your brand can also be a great addition, adding personality to your product and reinforcing the brand experience.

Packaging Solutions: Protecting and Presenting Your Products

Thoughtful packaging is essential for ensuring the safe transport of your products and effectively showcasing your brand to customers.

1. Durable, Attractive Packaging That Protects the Product During Transport Whether you are selling at a local market or shipping products across the country, it's crucial to choose packaging that will keep your items safe and in good condition.

   - For Soap and Lotion Bars: Packaging like kraft paper wraps, cardboard boxes, or tin containers provides durability while maintaining a natural, artisanal feel.

   - For Bath Bombs and Salts: Consider using glass jars, clear plastic containers, or eco-friendly kraft paper bags. These materials protect delicate products and give them an elegant appearance.

   - For Lip Balms: Small metal tins or sturdy plastic tubes are excellent choices to ensure the balm remains intact during transit.

2. Sustainable Options That Appeal to Eco-Conscious Consumers Offering eco-friendly packaging options shows that your brand cares about the environment and appeals to the growing number of sustainability-minded consumers.

- Recyclable Materials: Choose materials like glass, recycled cardboard, and biodegradable plastics.

- Minimalist Packaging: Use fewer plastic materials or go plastic-free whenever possible, opting for sustainable alternatives like compostable wraps or paper-based products.

- Refillable Options: Consider offering refillable packaging or reusable containers for products like lotion bars or bath salts, appealing to customers who want to minimize waste.

Scaling Up for Business: Growing Your Goat Milk Product Venture

As your goat milk product line gains popularity, scaling your business requires strategic planning across various fronts. By refining your pricing strategy and leveraging effective selling techniques, you can maximize your product's reach and profitability, driving the growth of your venture. Here's how to expand your business successfully.

Pricing Strategies

Establishing the right pricing strategy is crucial to ensure profitability while remaining competitive in the market.

1. Calculating Costs and Setting Competitive Prices: Pricing your products appropriately ensures that you cover production costs, make a profit, and remain competitive within your niche.

- Cost of Materials: Calculate the cost of ingredients, such as goat milk powder, essential oils, and carrier oils. Don't forget the packaging and labeling costs.

- Labor Costs: Consider your time spent creating the products—whether you're crafting them yourself or hiring help.

- Overhead Expenses: Include any costs for utilities, equipment, and space rental, if applicable.

- Market Research: Study your competitors' pricing to ensure that your prices are in line with industry standards while reflecting the quality and uniqueness of your products.

2. Offering Bundle Discounts for Gift Sets: Bundling products together at a discount can increase sales while offering added value to customers. It's also an excellent strategy for attracting gift-givers.

- Pre-made Bundles: Create themed bundles such as relaxation sets or spa packages that combine your bath bombs, soaps, lotions, and other products at a slightly discounted price.

- Seasonal Offers: Tailor bundles for holidays or special events like Christmas, Mother's Day, or Valentine's Day. These special sets are perfect for gifts and can encourage larger purchases.

- Discounts for Volume: Offer discounts for bulk purchases (e.g., buy two lotions, get one 10% off). This is an effective way to increase sales while providing customers with a great deal.

Marketing and Selling Tips

Building a strong brand presence and effectively reaching your target market is essential to scaling your goat milk product business.

1. Leveraging Social Media to Showcase Products and Engage with Customers: Social media platforms provide an excellent opportunity to engage with your audience, showcase your products, and build brand awareness.

   - High-Quality Visual Content: Post beautiful images of your products in use, showing their benefits and aesthetics. Share behind-the-scenes glimpses of the production process to build transparency and trust.

   - Engaging Posts: Create polls, ask questions, or share customer testimonials to interact with your followers. User-generated content, like customers' photos or reviews, can help build social proof.

   - Hashtags: Use relevant hashtags (#goatmilkproducts, #naturalbeauty, #handmadecosmetics) to increase discoverability and reach potential customers.

   - Influencer Partnerships: Collaborate with influencers or micro-influencers who align with your brand to reach a broader audience.

2. Participating in Local Craft Fairs and Farmers' Markets: In-person sales can help build local recognition and foster a loyal

customer base, especially for handmade products like goat milk soaps and lotions.

- **Booth Setup:** Design an inviting and professional booth that displays your products attractively. Offer free samples or demonstrations so potential customers can experience the products firsthand.

- **Personal Connection:** Engage with customers by sharing the story behind your brand and the benefits of goat milk-based products. Building relationships with customers in person can increase brand loyalty.

- **Offer Promotions:** Special event discounts, giveaways, or loyalty programs for repeat customers can help increase sales and encourage word-of-mouth referrals.

3. **Creating an Online Store or Partnering with Local Boutiques:** Expanding your reach beyond local markets allows you to access a global customer base and increase your sales potential.

- **Online Store:** Build an easy-to-navigate website or use e-commerce platforms like Etsy or Shopify to sell your products online. Include high-quality photos, clear descriptions, and straightforward checkout options.

- **Local Partnerships:** Reach out to local boutiques, gift shops, or home gift shops to see if they would be interested in carrying your products. Consignment deals or wholesale agreements can be a great way to get your products into stores.

- **Email Marketing:** Capture customer emails and send regular newsletters with updates, promotions, and new product releases. This helps keep customers engaged and encourages repeat purchases.

By implementing these marketing and selling strategies, you can effectively promote your goat milk products, enhance brand awareness, and grow your customer base.

This chapter offers a practical guide to creating high-quality, nourishing goat milk-based products, ideal for personal use, gifting, or launching a small business venture. Exploring the versatile benefits of goat milk, the chapter delves into a wide range of formulations, from soothing bath bombs and rejuvenating bath salts to hydrating lotion bars and nourishing lip balms.

Readers will find easy-to-follow recipes, along with customization tips for scents and textures, empowering them to craft personalized products tailored to individual preferences and skin types. The chapter also provides valuable insights on packaging and labeling, ensuring the final products are both visually appealing and safe for use or sale.

Goat milk is widely recognized for its exceptional nutritional profile and skin-nourishing properties, making it an ideal ingredient for a variety of personal care and beauty products. As the dairy goat sector continues to grow globally, the demand for high-quality goat milk-based offerings has also increased, presenting opportunities for entrepreneurs and hobbyists alike.

For those interested in turning their creations into a small business, the chapter covers essential aspects of pricing strategies, marketing techniques, and scaling up production to meet growing demand. Readers will learn how to effectively price their products, leverage diverse sales channels, and implement strategic marketing approaches to build brand recognition and reach a wider customer base.

Whether the goal is personal enjoyment or the launch of a successful entrepreneurial venture, this chapter equips readers with the knowledge and practical guidance to craft luxurious, natural goat milk products that can enhance skincare routines and become thoughtful, customized gifts or a thriving small business.

⤳

Chapter Nine:
Following Regulations, Guidelines, and Marketing Your Soap in Canada

Section 1: Understanding the Regulatory Framework for Selling Goat Milk Soap in Canada

Overview of Cosmetic Regulations in Canada

When it comes to selling goat milk soap in Canada, understanding the regulatory framework established by Health Canada is crucial. This governing body ensures that cosmetics sold within the country are safe for use and properly labeled. Goat milk soap, while often perceived as a natural or handmade product, is classified under Canadian law as a cosmetic.

According to Health Canada, a cosmetic is defined as:

"Any substance or mixture of substances manufactured, sold, or represented for use in cleansing, improving, or altering the complexion, skin, hair, or teeth."

This definition includes products like goat milk soap, which means they are subject to the same regulations as commercially manufactured skincare products.

Distinction Between Cosmetics and Natural Health Products (NHPs)

It is important to differentiate between cosmetics and natural health products (NHPs).

- Cosmetics are intended solely for external application to cleanse, beautify, or enhance appearance.

- NHPs, on the other hand, are products that claim therapeutic benefits, such as healing skin conditions or treating acne.

If your goat milk soap claims to have medicinal or therapeutic benefits—such as "healing eczema" or "reducing inflammation"—it may be reclassified as an NHP. This reclassification entails more stringent regulations, including clinical testing and licensing through the Natural and Non-prescription Health Products Directorate (NNHPD). Therefore, it is advisable to avoid making therapeutic claims unless you are prepared to comply with NHP regulations.

Role of the Food and Drugs Act and the Cosmetic Regulations

The sale of goat milk soap in Canada falls under the Food and Drugs Act and its associated Cosmetic Regulations. These regulations ensure that:

- Products are safe for human use.

- Ingredients are accurately disclosed.

- Labeling is clear and not misleading.

Compliance with these regulations not only ensures legal operation but also builds consumer trust by demonstrating a commitment to quality and transparency.

Legal Requirements for Labeling

Proper labeling of goat milk soap is essential for compliance with Canadian regulations and providing consumers with the necessary information to make informed purchasing decisions. Health Canada outlines specific requirements for both mandatory and optional label elements.

Mandatory Label Elements

Product Name: The label must display the product's common name, such as "Goat Milk Soap," along with the INCI (International Nomenclature of Cosmetic Ingredients) names for all ingredients. For example, goat milk should be listed as "Caprae Lac."

- Net Quantity: The net quantity of the product must be clearly displayed in metric units (grams or milliliters) on the front of the package. For instance, "100 g" or "250 ml."

- Name and Address of the Manufacturer or Distributor: The label must include the full name and address of the manufacturer or distributor responsible for the product, allowing consumers and regulatory authorities to contact the company if necessary.

- Language Requirements: Canada mandates bilingual labeling. All mandatory information must be provided in both English and French, ensuring accessibility to consumers across the country. For example: "Soap / Savon", "Net Weight / Poids Net".

- Warnings and Precautions: Any necessary warnings or precautions must be clearly stated on the label. For instance, if the product contains essential oils that may cause skin irritation, a label might read: "Warning: Contains essential oils. Perform a patch test before use."

Optional Label Elements

1. Claims About the Product's Benefits: While it may be tempting to highlight the benefits of goat milk soap, such as "moisturizing" or "nourishing," these claims must be carefully worded to comply with Health Canada regulations. Cosmetic claims should focus on general benefits like hydration or cleansing, rather than therapeutic outcomes. Acceptable claims might include: "Helps maintain soft, healthy skin" or "Gently cleanses without stripping natural oils."

2. Eco-Friendly or Organic Labels and Certifications: If your product is marketed as eco-friendly or organic, ensure that these claims are backed by legitimate certifications. Common certifications in Canada include EcoCert for

organic cosmetics and Leaping Bunny for cruelty-free products. Misleading environmental claims, known as greenwashing, can lead to regulatory action and damage your brand's reputation.

Key Considerations for Label Compliance

- **Legibility:** Labels must be easy to read, with clear fonts and sufficient contrast.

- **Durability:** Labels should be designed to withstand the environment in which the product will be used, such as humid bathrooms.

- **Ingredient Transparency:** Consumers are increasingly interested in knowing what goes into the products they use. Providing detailed ingredient information can enhance consumer trust and loyalty.

Section 2: Registering Products with Health Canada

Introduction to the Cosmetic Notification Form (CNF)

Before you can sell goat milk soap in Canada, it is essential to register your product with Health Canada by submitting a Cosmetic Notification Form (CNF). This process is mandatory for all cosmetic products under the Cosmetic Regulations of the Food and Drugs Act.

The CNF serves to provide Health Canada with detailed information about your cosmetic product, ensuring its compliance with safety regulations and confirming that it does not pose any health risks to consumers. Submitting a CNF also enables Health Canada to monitor products on the market and take regulatory action if any safety issues arise.

Why Is the CNF Mandatory?

- It ensures transparency and traceability for all cosmetic products sold in Canada.

- It allows Health Canada to maintain a database of cosmetics for consumer safety and product recalls.

- Non-compliance can lead to enforcement actions, such as product recalls, fines, or bans on sales.

Timeline and Steps for Submitting the Form

Once you decide to sell your goat milk soap, the CNF must be submitted within 10 days of your product being made available for sale. To avoid delays, it is advisable to submit the CNF as soon as the product formulation and labeling are finalized.

Step-by-Step Guide to Registering Your Product

1. Creating an Account with the Cosmetics Program

To initiate the registration process, you need to create an account with Health Canada's Cosmetics Program through the online submission portal.

- Visit the Health Canada Cosmetic Notification website.

- Register for an account by providing your personal or business information, including the name and address of the manufacturer or distributor.

- Once your account is verified, you can log in to access the CNF submission platform.

2. Completing the CNF

The Cosmetic Notification Form requires specific information about your product. Ensure all details are accurate and up-to-date.

- Product Classification: Identify the product category (e.g., bar soap, liquid soap) and confirm that your goat milk soap falls under the cosmetic classification, not as a natural health product.

- Detailed List of Ingredients and Concentrations: Provide a comprehensive list of all ingredients using their INCI (International Nomenclature of Cosmetic Ingredients) names, specifying the concentration of each ingredient in percentage form. For example: Caprae Lac (Goat Milk)–10%.

- Purpose and Intended Use of the Product: Clearly state the product's intended cosmetic use. For instance: "This soap is intended for cleansing and moisturizing the skin."

- Safety Data Sheets (SDS): If your product contains chemicals or ingredients that require safety documentation, attach the relevant Safety Data Sheets (SDS). These sheets provide information on handling, storage, and potential hazards. While goat milk soap made from natural ingredients may not always require SDS, certain essential oils or preservatives might.

3. Submitting the CNF

- Review all the information in the CNF to ensure accuracy and completeness.

- Submit the CNF through the online portal.

- You will receive a confirmation email once the form is successfully submitted. Keep this confirmation for your records.

Managing Product Notifications for New Batches or Formulations

Whenever you introduce a new batch, modify the formulation, or change the product label, you must update the CNF to reflect these changes.

- New Formulation: Submit a new CNF if you significantly change the ingredients or their concentrations.

- Batch Notification: While individual batches do not require notification, any safety concerns or product recalls must be reported.

Staying Compliant

Updating Notifications for Product Changes

It is crucial to keep your CNF up-to-date to remain compliant with Health Canada's regulations. This includes:

- Updating the CNF if you change suppliers or the sourcing of raw materials.

- Notifying Health Canada if you discontinue the product or make significant changes to the packaging or labeling.

Record-Keeping

Maintaining accurate records is essential for compliance and smooth operation. These records should include:

- Copies of all CNF submissions and updates.

- Ingredient sourcing information, including supplier details and batch numbers.

- Production dates and batch-specific data for traceability.

- Safety data sheets for ingredients with potential hazards.

Availability of Documentation During Inspections

Health Canada may conduct routine inspections or investigations in response to consumer complaints. During these inspections, you may be required to provide:

- Copies of CNF submissions.

- Records of ingredient sourcing and supplier information.

- Documentation of manufacturing practices and batch production details.

Failure to provide the required documentation during an inspection can lead to penalties, including fines or product recalls.

Section 3: Importance of Documentation

Proper documentation is essential for the success and compliance of your goat milk soap business. Not only does it ensure adherence to Health Canada regulations, but it also fosters consumer trust, enhances product safety, and streamlines operations. This section will explore key documentation practices that every soap manufacturer should follow.

Ingredient Documentation

Maintaining accurate and detailed records of all ingredients used in your goat milk soap is crucial for transparency, traceability, and compliance.

1. Sourcing Records

Keeping comprehensive sourcing records allows you to verify the quality and safety of your ingredients, ensuring consistency in product formulation.

- Supplier Information: Document the name, address, and contact details of each supplier.

- Ingredient Specifications: Record the INCI name, common name, and purity level of each ingredient.

- Certificates of Analysis (COA): Request COAs from suppliers to confirm the quality and safety of raw materials.

- Lot or Batch Numbers: Track lot or batch numbers for each ingredient to maintain traceability.

2. Safety and Allergen Documentation

Ingredient safety is critical, especially for consumers with allergies or sensitivities.

- Safety Data Sheets (SDS): Retain SDS for all chemical or hazardous ingredients used, even if they are derived from natural sources.

- Allergen Information: Document potential allergens, such as essential oils or preservatives, and ensure they are clearly listed on product labels.

- Preservative Efficacy Testing: If using preservatives, maintain records of efficacy tests to ensure they provide adequate protection against microbial growth.

Production Records

Accurate production records are vital for quality control, consistency, and traceability in case of a product recall or safety concern.

3. Tracking Production Dates and Batch Numbers

Assign unique batch numbers to each production run to track products from manufacturing to sale.

- Production Date: Record the date each batch was produced.

- Batch Number: Assign a batch number that corresponds to production details, including ingredient sources and quantities.

- Production Quantity: Document the total number of units produced in each batch.

4. Developing a Traceability System

A traceability system ensures that you can quickly identify and address any issues related to a specific batch.

- Batch Tracking: Implement a system that links each batch to its ingredients, production date, and distribution channels.

- Recall Procedures: Develop a recall plan outlining steps for identifying affected batches, notifying customers, and removing products from the market.

Storage and Expiration Records

Proper storage and monitoring of expiration dates are essential for maintaining the quality and safety of your goat milk soap.

5. Proper Storage Conditions

Goat milk soap contains natural ingredients that may be sensitive to environmental conditions.

- Temperature: Store soap in a cool, dry place to prevent melting or spoilage.

- Humidity: Minimize exposure to humidity to prevent mold growth and maintain product integrity.

- Packaging: Use airtight packaging to protect soap from contaminants and extend its shelf life.

6. Monitoring Shelf Life

Tracking the shelf life of your goat milk soap is essential for ensuring product safety and effectiveness.

- Expiration Dates: Assign a shelf life based on ingredient stability and preservative efficacy.

- Rotation System: Implement a first-in, first-out (FIFO) system to ensure older products are sold before newer ones.

- Periodic Inspections: Regularly inspect stored products for signs of spoilage, such as discoloration, odor changes, or mold growth.

7. Managing Expired Products

Expired products should be removed from inventory to prevent them from reaching consumers.

- Disposal Records: Maintain records of expired products and their disposal methods.

- Inventory Adjustments: Update inventory records to reflect the removal of expired products.

Benefits of Maintaining Proper Documentation

- Regulatory Compliance: Documentation helps you adhere to Health Canada's Cosmetic Regulations and facilitates smooth inspections.

- Consumer Trust: Transparent records and accurate labeling build trust with customers, enhancing your brand reputation.

- Quality Control: Detailed production and storage records ensure consistent product quality and safety.

- Efficient Recalls: A robust traceability system allows for quick and effective product recalls, minimizing the impact on your business and customers.

Section 4: Exploring Sales Venues for Goat Milk Soap

Selling goat milk soap presents a variety of opportunities across different sales venues, each with its unique advantages and challenges. By diversifying your sales channels—whether through face-to-face interactions or the convenience of online platforms—you can expand your customer base and grow your business effectively.

Craft Sales and Farmers' Markets

Local craft fairs and farmers' markets are excellent venues for selling handmade goat milk soap, particularly for small-scale producers aiming to establish a community presence.

Benefits of Selling at Local Markets

- Direct Customer Interaction: Build relationships with customers, receive immediate feedback, and gain insights into their preferences.

- Brand Visibility: Increase brand recognition within your local community.

- Low Marketing Costs: Leverage word-of-mouth marketing and the market's existing customer base.

Tips for Applying and Securing Vendor Spots

Research Local Events: Identify craft fairs and farmers' markets that attract your target audience.

- Early Application: Apply early, as vendor spots can fill quickly, especially for popular markets.

- Prepare a Portfolio: Include photos of your products, booth setup, and any branding materials to enhance your application.

- Vendor Requirements: Review each market's guidelines regarding product types, booth sizes, and fees.

Setting Up an Attractive and Engaging Booth Display

- Visual Appeal: Use clean, well-organized displays with attractive signage that highlights key product features, such as "handmade," "organic," or "locally sourced."

- Branding: Incorporate your brand colors, logo, and packaging to create a cohesive look.

- Interactive Elements: Offer product samples or demonstrations to engage customers.

- Pricing and Promotions: Clearly display prices and consider offering bundle deals or discounts for multiple purchases.

- Comfort and Accessibility: Provide a welcoming space with ample lighting, comfortable flooring, and easy access for all customers.

Consignment Shops and Local Retailers

Partnering with local boutiques and gift shops can help expand your market reach and attract customers who appreciate artisanal, locally made products.

Approaching Local Boutiques and Gift Shops

- Research Potential Partners: Identify shops that align with your brand and target audience.

- Professional Pitch: Prepare a professional pitch that includes product samples, a business card, and a product catalog or price sheet.

- Highlight Unique Selling Points: Emphasize what sets your goat milk soap apart, such as natural ingredients, eco-friendly packaging, or community involvement.

Negotiating Consignment Agreements and Wholesale Pricing

Consignment vs. Wholesale:

- Consignment: The retailer pays you after the product is sold, which is common for small businesses.

- Wholesale: The retailer buys your products upfront at a discounted rate.

Key Agreement Terms:

- Payment Terms: Specify payment schedules and percentages for consignment sales.

- Product Display: Outline how and where your products will be displayed.

- Inventory Management: Agree on how inventory levels will be tracked and restocked.

- Returns and Damages: Clarify who is responsible for unsold or damaged products.

Online Sales Platforms

Expanding to online sales allows you to reach customers beyond your local area and operate your business with greater flexibility.

Setting Up an E-Commerce Store

Platform Selection: Choose an e-commerce platform that suits your needs, such as:

- Shopify: Ideal for creating a standalone online store with customizable features.

- Etsy: A popular marketplace for handmade and artisanal products with an existing customer base.

- Amazon Handmade: Provides access to Amazon's vast customer network but requires compliance with specific guidelines.

Product Listings:

- High-Quality Photos: Use clear, well-lit images that showcase your soap from multiple angles.

- Detailed Descriptions: Include information about ingredients, benefits, and usage instructions.

- SEO Optimization: Use relevant keywords to improve search visibility and attract potential customers.

Pricing Strategy:

- Factor in production costs, platform fees, and shipping costs.

- Research competitor pricing to ensure your products remain competitive while maintaining profitability.

Shipping Logistics and Costs in Canada and Internationally

Domestic Shipping:

- Partner with reliable shipping carriers like Canada Post, Purolator, or FedEx.

- Offer flat-rate or free shipping for orders over a certain amount to encourage larger purchases.

International Shipping:

- Understand customs regulations and documentation requirements for international shipments.

- Clearly communicate shipping timelines, costs, and potential duties or taxes to customers.

- Offer tracking and insurance for international orders to ensure a positive customer experience.

Packaging for Shipping:

- Use sturdy, eco-friendly packaging that protects products during transit.

- Include branded inserts, such as thank-you notes or care instructions, to enhance customer satisfaction.

Combining Sales Channels for Maximum Impact

Diversifying your sales channels—by combining in-person markets, retail partnerships, and online platforms—can maximize your reach and profitability. Each channel offers unique opportunities to engage with customers and showcase your goat milk soap in different ways.

Section 5: Developing a Successful Marketing Strategy

An effective marketing strategy is crucial for building brand awareness, attracting customers, and driving sales for your goat milk soap business. By establishing a strong brand identity, creating compliant and appealing product labels, and utilizing various marketing channels, you can position your products for success in a competitive marketplace.

Creating a Brand Identity

Your brand identity serves as the foundation of your marketing strategy, influencing how customers perceive your business and products.

Choosing a Business Name and Logo

Business Name:

- Reflect your product's key attributes, such as natural, organic, or handmade.

- Keep it simple, memorable, and easy to pronounce.

- Consider including "goat milk" or "soap" in the name for clarity.

- Check for domain name availability to ensure consistency across online platforms.

Logo Design:

- Work with a professional graphic designer or use design tools like Canva or Adobe Express.

- Choose colors and fonts that align with your brand's personality (e.g., earthy tones for a natural brand or elegant fonts for a luxury product).

- Ensure the logo is versatile and works well on labels, packaging, and digital platforms.

Defining Your Brand's Core Values and Mission

Core Values:

- Sustainability: Emphasize eco-friendly practices, such as using biodegradable packaging and sourcing ethically produced ingredients.

- Quality: Highlight the handmade nature of your soap and the benefits of using goat milk.

- Community: Showcase your involvement in local events or charitable initiatives.

Mission Statement:

- Craft a concise statement that communicates your brand's purpose and what sets it apart from competitors.

Example: "Our mission is to provide natural, nourishing skincare products that promote healthy skin while supporting sustainable and ethical practices."

Designing Effective Product Labels

Product labels are a critical touchpoint for customers, serving both functional and marketing purposes.

Eye-Catching Designs That Comply with Canadian Labeling Laws

Compliance:

- Include all mandatory information as required by Health Canada, such as product name, ingredient list, net quantity, and manufacturer details in both English and French.

- Ensure font size, color contrast, and layout are clear and easy to read.

Design Elements:

- Use high-quality images and graphics that reflect your brand's identity.

- Incorporate texture, embossing, or metallic finishes for a premium look.

- Choose materials that align with your brand values, such as recycled or biodegradable label stock.

Including QR Codes for Digital Interaction

Purpose of QR Codes:

- Link to your website, online store, or social media pages.

- Provide access to product information, ingredient details, or instructional videos.

- Encourage customers to leave reviews or sign up for your newsletter.

Placement:

- Position the QR code in a visible but unobtrusive spot on the label.

- Test the code to ensure it scans correctly and leads to the intended destination.

Leveraging Social Media for Promotion

Social media platforms are powerful tools for building brand awareness, engaging with customers, and driving traffic to your online store.

Identifying the Best Platforms for Your Audience

- Instagram: Perfect for sharing visually appealing content and connecting with beauty and skincare enthusiasts.

- Facebook: Effective for building a community, sharing updates, and running targeted ads.

- TikTok: Great for reaching younger audiences and showcasing creative, short-form videos.

- Pinterest: Useful for driving traffic to your website through visually engaging pins.

Strategies for Posting Engaging Content

Behind-the-Scenes Content:

- Share photos and videos of the soap-making process, ingredient sourcing, and packaging.

- Highlight the craftsmanship and care that goes into each product.

Customer Testimonials and Reviews:

- Feature positive feedback from customers to build trust and credibility.

- Encourage customers to tag your brand in their posts and share user-generated content.

Educational Posts:

- Create content that educates your audience on the benefits of goat milk soap, such as its moisturizing properties, gentle cleansing, and suitability for sensitive skin.

- Offer skincare tips, DIY recipes, or ingredient spotlights to position yourself as an authority in natural skincare.

Consistent Posting Schedule:

- Develop a content calendar to plan and schedule posts in advance.

- Use tools like Hootsuite, Buffer, or Later to automate posting and track engagement.

Email Marketing and Newsletters

Email marketing is a cost-effective way to stay connected with your customers, promote new products, and drive repeat sales.

Building an Email List

Sign-Up Forms:

- Add sign-up forms to your website, online store, and social media profiles.

- Offer incentives for subscribing, such as a discount code, free sample, or exclusive content.

In-Person Collection:

- Collect email addresses at craft fairs, farmers' markets, and other events.

- Use a tablet or paper sign-up sheet, providing a clear explanation of the benefits of joining your list.

Sending Regular Updates, Promotions, and Product Launches

Newsletter Content:

- Share company news, behind-the-scenes stories, and customer testimonials.

- Announce new product launches, seasonal promotions, and upcoming events.

- Include links to your online store, social media pages, and blog.

Personalization and Segmentation:

- Personalize emails with the recipient's name and tailor content based on their purchase history or interests.

- Segment your email list to send targeted messages to different customer groups, such as first-time buyers, repeat customers, or VIP members.

Email Design:

- Use a clean, visually appealing layout that reflects your brand's identity.

- Ensure emails are mobile-friendly and include clear calls to action (e.g., "Shop Now," "Learn More," or "Leave a Review").

Section 6: Building and Nurturing a Customer Base

A loyal customer base is vital for long-term success in the goat milk soap industry. By building strong relationships, engaging with the community, and providing excellent customer service, you can create repeat customers and brand advocates.

Networking and Community Engagement

Developing meaningful connections with local businesses, influencers, and the community can significantly enhance your brand's visibility and credibility.

Collaborating with Local Businesses

Joint Promotions:

- Partner with complementary businesses, such as spas, salons, or health food stores, to offer bundled products or cross-promotions.

- Host joint events or workshops that showcase both your products and their services.

Pop-Up Shops:

- Set up temporary retail spaces in local boutiques, coffee shops, or community centers.

- Leverage the existing customer base of these businesses to introduce your products to new audiences.

Participating in Community Events

Local Fairs and Festivals:

- Attend events that align with your target audience, such as wellness expos, artisan markets, or eco-friendly festivals.

- Use these opportunities to network with other vendors, meet potential customers, and gather valuable feedback.

Charity and Fundraising Events:

- Donate a portion of your sales or provide gift baskets for local fundraisers and charity events.

- This not only supports a good cause but also positions your brand as socially responsible and community-oriented.

Partnering with Influencers or Local Personalities

Micro-Influencers:

- Collaborate with influencers who have a small but engaged following within your niche.

- Offer free products in exchange for honest reviews, social media posts, or blog features.

Local Ambassadors:

- Identify well-known community figures or small business owners who align with your brand values.

- Provide them with exclusive products and discounts to promote your brand within their network.

Providing Excellent Customer Service

Exceptional customer service is key to building trust, loyalty, and positive word-of-mouth for your brand.

Handling Customer Inquiries and Complaints Professionally:

- Timely Responses: Aim to respond to customer inquiries within 24 hours, whether via email, social media, or phone. Use automated responses to acknowledge receipt of inquiries and set expectations for follow-up.

- Empathetic Communication: Listen to customer concerns with empathy and understanding. Offer clear solutions and, when appropriate, provide compensation such as discounts, refunds, or replacements.

- Clear Policies: Establish and communicate clear policies for returns, exchanges, and refunds. Ensure your policies are easily accessible on your website and printed materials.

Offering Personalized Recommendations:

- Understanding Customer Needs: Ask questions to understand customers' skin types, concerns, and preferences. Recommend specific products or combinations that best suit their needs.

- Follow-up: Reach out to customers after their purchase to ensure they are satisfied with their products. Offer additional tips or suggestions for product use and care.

Collecting and Utilizing Customer Feedback

Feedback from customers is invaluable for improving your products, customer experience, and overall business operations.

Encouraging Reviews and Testimonials:

- Requesting Reviews: Encourage customers to leave reviews on your website, social media pages, or third-party platforms like Google or Yelp. Offer incentives such as discounts or entry into a giveaway for submitting a review.

- Displaying Testimonials: Highlight positive customer testimonials on your website, product packaging, and marketing materials. Use photos and quotes to add authenticity and credibility.

Using Feedback to Improve Products and Customer Experience:

- Product Development: Analyze feedback to identify common themes or issues, such as scent preferences, packaging functionality, or skin reactions. Use this information to refine existing products or develop new ones that better meet customer needs.

- Customer Experience: Evaluate feedback related to the purchasing process, shipping times, or customer service interactions. Implement changes to streamline and enhance the customer experience, such as improving website navigation, offering faster shipping options, or providing more detailed product descriptions.

Building Customer Loyalty

Show appreciation for feedback by publicly acknowledging customer suggestions and implementing improvements. Engage with customers on social media, respond to their comments, and build a community around your brand.

Section 7: Personal Experiences and Lessons Learned

Every entrepreneurial journey is marked by both successes and challenges. Sharing personal experiences can provide invaluable insights for those navigating the path of selling goat milk soap in Canada. This section explores real-life stories, lessons learned, and strategies for overcoming obstacles in the natural skincare industry.

Success Stories from Craft Fairs

Participating in craft fairs and farmers' markets has been crucial for building a loyal customer base and enhancing visibility within the community.

Memorable Customer Interactions

- **First-Time Customers Turned Regulars:** One of the most rewarding experiences was a customer who initially bought a single bar of soap as a gift. Weeks later, they returned excitedly to share how much the recipient loved the product's moisturizing effects. This interaction blossomed into a long-term relationship, with the customer becoming a regular and recommending the soap to friends and family.

- **Building Community Relationships:** A local artisan who shared a booth at a holiday market became a significant partner for cross-promotions. Their handmade candles complemented the goat milk soap perfectly, leading to co-hosted events and increased sales for both businesses.

Lessons Learned from Craft Fairs

- **The Importance of Presentation:** A visually appealing booth with clear branding, well-arranged products, and engaging signage consistently attracted more foot traffic. Investing in a professional-looking display and incorporating live demonstrations or samples significantly boosted sales.

- **Customer Engagement is Key:** Engaging with potential customers by sharing the story behind the brand and offering personalized recommendations often led to higher conversion rates. It became evident that customers were drawn to authenticity and transparency.

Challenges Faced in the Market

The natural skincare industry is highly competitive and constantly evolving, presenting unique challenges for small business owners.

Navigating Competition

- **Standing Out in a Crowded Market:** Competing against well-established brands and other local artisans required a focus on product differentiation. Emphasizing the unique qualities of the goat milk soap—such as locally sourced ingredients, eco-friendly packaging, and handcrafted quality—helped carve out a niche in the market.

- Leveraging Customer Loyalty: While attracting new customers is crucial, retaining existing ones proved equally important. Implementing a customer loyalty program, offering discounts for referrals, and maintaining consistent communication through email newsletters helped sustain repeat business.

Dealing with Regulatory Changes

- Staying Informed: Keeping up with changes in cosmetic regulations and Health Canada's requirements was an ongoing challenge. Subscribing to regulatory updates and joining industry associations provided timely information and resources to ensure compliance.

- Adapting to New Requirements: When new labeling guidelines were introduced, it necessitated a significant investment in redesigning packaging. However, the updated labels, which featured clearer ingredient lists and bilingual instructions, ultimately improved the product's marketability.

Growth and Expansion

Expanding a local goat milk soap business into new markets requires strategic planning and a willingness to adapt.

Tips for Scaling Your Business

- Investing in Production: Scaling production from small batches to larger quantities involved upgrading equipment, sourcing ingredients in bulk, and streamlining processes without compromising quality. Documenting standard operating procedures (SOPs) ensured consistency and efficiency.

- Building a Team: Hiring part-time staff for production, packaging, and customer service allowed the business to focus on growth and marketing efforts. Training employees on brand values and product knowledge was essential for maintaining a cohesive customer experience.

Exploring Export Opportunities and International Sales

- Researching Export Markets: Expanding beyond Canada involved researching international markets with a demand for natural and organic skincare products. Countries with a growing interest in eco-friendly and handmade goods, such as the United States and Europe, became primary targets.

- Navigating Export Regulations: Exporting cosmetic products requires understanding the regulations of the destination country, including labeling, packaging, and product safety standards. Partnering with international distributors and attending trade shows helped facilitate the expansion process.

- Leveraging E-Commerce: Establishing an online store with international shipping options allowed the brand to reach customers worldwide. Collaborating with fulfillment centers and optimizing shipping logistics ensured timely and cost-effective deliveries.

Section 8: Additional Resources

A successful goat milk soap business depends not only on product quality and effective marketing but also on staying informed, connected, and committed to continuous improvement. This section provides a curated list of regulatory bodies, support organizations, educational resources, and workshops that can assist entrepreneurs in navigating the industry and growing their businesses.

Regulatory Bodies and Support Organizations

Understanding industry standards and ensuring compliance with regulations is crucial for long-term success. The following organizations offer valuable guidance, resources, and support for cosmetic businesses in Canada.

1. Health Canada's Cosmetics Program

Website: Health Canada Cosmetics Program

Health Canada regulates cosmetics, including goat milk soap. The Cosmetics Program website provides essential information on:

- Cosmetic Notification Forms (CNFs) and submission guidelines.

- Updates on labeling and safety requirements.

- Guidance documents and FAQs for cosmetic manufacturers.

2. Canadian Cosmetic, Toiletry, and Fragrance Association (CCTFA)

Website: CCTFA

The CCTFA is a leading trade association representing the cosmetic and personal care products industry in Canada. Membership benefits include:

- Access to industry news and regulatory updates.

- Networking opportunities with other cosmetic manufacturers and suppliers.

- Educational webinars and training sessions on compliance and best practices.

Local Health Authorities

Provincial and municipal health authorities may impose additional regulations regarding the sale of handmade cosmetics at local events and farmers' markets. Maintaining communication with these agencies can help ensure compliance with local bylaws and inspection requirements.

Educational Resources and Workshops

Continuous learning is key to staying competitive and enhancing the quality of your products. The following resources offer training, certifications, and business development opportunities.

Online Courses and Certification Programs for Soap-Making

Several online platforms provide comprehensive courses in soap-making, covering topics from basic techniques to advanced formulations.

- Handcrafted Soap & Cosmetic Guild (HSCG): Offers online and in-person workshops, certification programs, and industry events.

- Soap Queen (Bramble Berry): Provides various video tutorials and blog posts on soap-making techniques, business tips, and product formulation.

- Udemy: Features a wide range of courses on natural skincare formulation, branding, and marketing for small businesses.

Business Development Programs and Local Chambers of Commerce

Entrepreneurs can benefit from local resources that support small businesses, including:

- Small Business Enterprise Centres (SBECs): Located in various cities across Canada, SBECs provide free consultations, workshops, and networking events for small business owners.

- Local Chambers of Commerce: Membership in a chamber of commerce opens doors to valuable networking opportunities, marketing resources, and mentorship programs.

- Women's Enterprise Organizations: For women entrepreneurs, organizations like the Women's Enterprise Centre offer tailored business advisory services, funding opportunities, and educational programs.

Industry Events and Trade Shows

Attending industry events and trade shows provides invaluable opportunities for learning, networking, and showcasing your products.

- Canadian Gift Association (CanGift) Fairs: These trade shows attract retailers and buyers looking for unique, handcrafted products, making them an excellent platform for expanding your market.

- Natural Health Product Expos: Events focused on natural and organic products provide insights into market trends, ingredient sourcing, and regulatory changes.

- Local Craft Fairs and Farmers' Markets: Participating in regional events not only boosts sales but also fosters relationships with other artisans and potential business partners.

By leveraging these resources, entrepreneurs can stay informed, build valuable connections, and continuously enhance their business. Whether you are just starting or looking to expand, the right tools and networks can significantly impact your journey to success.

∾

Chapter Ten:
Conclusion

The journey of making goat milk soap is both rewarding and transformative, evolving from simple beginnings into a deeply personal and creative pursuit. Initially, there's a mix of curiosity and hesitation as you navigate this new territory. Understanding the core ingredients—goat milk, lye, and natural oils—along with mastering essential techniques like proper mixing, curing, and safety protocols lays the groundwork for success. While these early steps may seem daunting, each challenge you overcome builds your confidence.

As you advance, soap-making shifts from a focus on following instructions to one of exploration and personalization. The thrill of experimenting with various scents, colors, and textures adds a creative layer to the process. Balancing the nourishing properties of goat milk with complementary ingredients such as essential oils, herbs, and clays opens up limitless possibilities. Over time, you refine your skills to craft not only functional products but also beautiful works of art that embody your unique style and vision.

The challenges you face—whether it's achieving the perfect consistency, troubleshooting unexpected results, or trying out new recipes—become invaluable learning experiences. Each obstacle fosters patience and resilience, deepening your understanding of the craft. These moments serve as reminders that growth often arises from the willingness to make mistakes and learn from them.

Encouragement to Embrace Creativity

Soap making is a vibrant canvas for boundless creativity, offering endless opportunities for experimentation and innovation. By exploring a variety of scents, colors, and molds, you can transform simple soap into a unique expression of your personality and style. Imagine crafting a calming lavender-scented soap shaped like flowers or creating a bold, multi-colored swirl design infused with invigorating citrus oils. These creative choices not only make your soaps stand out but also provide a deeply satisfying outlet for artistic expression.

Engaging in creativity while making soap opens doors to new ideas and inspirations. You might develop a signature blend that becomes your hallmark or invent a novel technique that others admire and replicate. This creative journey extends beyond soap—perhaps you'll design packaging that reflects your personality or create themed gift sets for holidays and special occasions.

Moreover, soap-making can spark new traditions. You might involve friends and family in crafting personalized soaps for celebrations, turning it into a cherished annual event. Seasonal creations, like pumpkin spice for autumn or peppermint swirls for winter, can become part of your holiday rituals, creating lasting memories with loved ones.

Beyond personal expression, the creativity found in soap-making fosters a sense of connection and individuality. Each unique bar reflects your passion and dedication, serving as a reminder of the joy and fulfillment that comes from transforming simple ingredients into something extraordinary.

Personal and Community Impact

There's an unparalleled joy that comes from creating something with your own hands. Soap-making, in particular, provides a deep sense of accomplishment and pride as you transform simple, natural ingredients into beautiful and functional products. The process of crafting your own soap fosters a connection to your work, allowing you to appreciate the effort and care that goes into each bar. It serves as a reminder of the value of handmade items in a world that often prioritizes convenience over craftsmanship.

Sharing these handmade creations enhances the satisfaction even further. Whether you gift a bar of soap to a friend, sell it at a local market, or offer it as a token of appreciation, the personal touch resonates with those who receive it. Handmade soaps carry a unique story—a narrative of thoughtfulness, effort, and care—that makes them far more meaningful than mass-produced alternatives.

Moreover, soap-making has the power to strengthen community bonds. Selling your soaps at local markets can be a wonderful way to connect with neighbors and cultivate relationships with customers who appreciate natural, handcrafted products. It becomes more than just a transaction; it's an opportunity to share your passion, exchange ideas, and inspire others to embrace sustainable and creative practices.

Hosting soap-making workshops is another excellent way to foster community spirit. By teaching others the craft, you not only spread knowledge but also create a collaborative space for camaraderie. Participants leave with new skills, a sense of accomplishment, and perhaps even new friendships.

Even small gestures, like exchanging soaps as gifts, can have a significant impact. A handmade soap tailored to someone's favorite scent or crafted with a personal touch speaks volumes about your thoughtfulness. These exchanges create moments of connection and gratitude that strengthen relationships and reinforce the sense of community.

Sustainability and Self-Sufficiency

One of the most compelling reasons to make soap at home is the positive impact it has on the environment. In a world where plastic packaging and synthetic chemicals are rampant, creating your own soap offers a meaningful way to reduce waste and promote sustainability. By choosing simple, natural ingredients and packaging your soap in reusable or recyclable containers, you significantly cut down on the plastic waste typically associated with store-bought products. This shift toward minimalistic, eco-friendly packaging is an easy yet effective way to contribute positively to reducing environmental harm.

Additionally, making homemade soap allows you to avoid the harmful chemicals commonly found in commercial products. Many commercial soaps contain synthetic fragrances, artificial colors, and preservatives that can be detrimental to both our health and the environment. By crafting your own soap, you have complete control over the ingredients you use, ensuring that your creations are free from harsh chemicals and toxins. This benefits not only your skin but also helps protect aquatic ecosystems by preventing harmful substances from entering the water supply.

Soap-making fits seamlessly into broader homesteading practices, which emphasize sustainability and self-sufficiency. For instance, if you raise goats on your homestead, you can use their milk to create nourishing, natural soap. This connection between the animals you care for and the products you create adds a fulfilling layer to the process, reinforcing a sense of responsibility and harmony with nature. The same principles apply if you grow your own herbs—such as lavender, chamomile, or calendula—for use in soap making, further reducing the need for store-bought ingredients.

Incorporating natural dyes into your soap recipes, like turmeric, spirulina, or beetroot powder, is another way to promote a sustainable lifestyle. These plant-based colors are gentle on the environment and provide a safe, eco-friendly alternative to synthetic dyes, which can be toxic and pollute waterways. By embracing these natural alternatives, you create soaps that are kind to both the skin and the earth.

Furthermore, soap-making encourages a deeper connection to the land and the resources available to you. It serves as a reminder of the power of self-sufficiency—an essential component of homesteading. Whether crafting soap from goat milk, harvesting herbs from your garden, or experimenting with sustainable packaging solutions, soap-making is a wonderful way to embrace a holistic, self-sustaining lifestyle.

Soap-Making as a Business Opportunity

Soap making is more than just a fulfilling hobby; it can also be a pathway to entrepreneurship. With a rising interest in natural, handmade products, there is a significant demand for high-quality soaps that truly stand out in the market. Here are some practical steps to help you turn your passion for soap making into a thriving business.

Branding and Marketing

The first step is to define your brand. What makes your soap unique? Is it the use of goat milk, all-natural ingredients, or a distinct aesthetic appeal? Create a unique name, logo, and packaging that reflects your vision and resonates with your target audience. Utilize online platforms like Instagram, Pinterest, and Etsy to showcase your products, telling the story behind each bar of soap and how it connects to sustainability and self-care.

Understanding Customer Needs

Research is crucial for success. Engage with potential customers to understand their preferences—whether they favor particular scents, have skin sensitivities, or value eco-friendly packaging. Consider offering samples at local markets or fairs to gather feedback and adjust your product offerings accordingly. Building a loyal customer base begins with listening to their needs and consistently delivering exceptional value.

Starting Small, Growing Gradually

Begin with small-scale production to refine your recipes and processes while keeping costs manageable. Focus on quality over quantity to establish a reputation for excellence. As demand increases, consider expanding your product line to include specialty items such as seasonal soaps, gift sets, or subscription boxes. Gradually scaling up allows you to maintain the authenticity and uniqueness that makes handmade soaps so special.

Building a Community

Connecting with like-minded artisans and customers helps foster a supportive network. Collaborate with local businesses, participate in craft fairs, or host workshops to share your expertise. These connections not only enhance your visibility but also strengthen your roots within the community, creating lasting relationships that support your business.

Starting a soap-making business offers endless potential for creativity, financial growth, and meaningful connections. With dedication, attention to detail, and a commitment to your values, you can turn your passion into a profitable and rewarding endeavor.

Acknowledgment of Reader's Growth

As you conclude this journey, take a moment to reflect on how far you've come. You've not only mastered the technical skills of soap making, but also developed a mindset geared toward experimentation, innovation, and growth. Whether this was your first batch or you've already crafted several dozen, each step has contributed to your personal development.

Celebrate Your Achievements

Every milestone in your soap-making journey—whether it's perfecting your first recipe or mastering intricate designs—deserves recognition. No achievement is too small to celebrate. Perhaps your soaps have improved in texture, scent, or appearance. Maybe you've gained the confidence to explore new techniques or ingredients. These accomplishments are a testament to your dedication and creativity, so take the time to celebrate them!

Skills Gained

Throughout this process, you've cultivated a diverse set of skills that will serve you well beyond soap making. Patience and attention to detail have been essential in crafting flawless products. You've learned to be resourceful, effectively handling unexpected challenges and adapting when things didn't go as planned. Most importantly, you've gained a profound understanding of sustainability, from sourcing natural ingredients to minimize packaging waste.

Additionally, you've explored the fundamentals of entrepreneurship, whether through small-scale sales or experimenting with different branding strategies. These skills are transferable, allowing you to venture into other creative businesses or simply enrich your lifestyle with practical, hands-on knowledge.

The Bigger Picture

The journey you've embarked on with soap making is just the beginning of a greater transformation—one that transcends the soap you create. It's about embracing a mindset of self-sufficiency, sustainability, and creativity in all areas of life. Whether you continue making soap for personal use, share it with friends and family, or decide to turn it into a business, you have laid the foundation for something meaningful.

Your growth as a soap maker is not solely about the end product, but also about the process and learning experiences that have shaped you. As you continue to experiment, refine your craft, and build your community, you will keep evolving in new and exciting ways. So, take pride in your accomplishments and remember that this journey is one of both personal and creative evolution.

Gratitude and Closing Message

As we reach the end of this book, I want to take a moment to express my heartfelt gratitude for your time, effort, and commitment. You've invested in yourself and your craft, taking the first steps toward creating something meaningful with your own hands. Whether you've been making soap for years or have just begun, the journey you've undertaken is one of growth, creativity, and connection. I hope this book has not only taught you the art of soap making but also inspired you to explore new ideas, embrace natural living, and share your creations with others.

Your decision to embark on this journey is a step toward something truly special—a community of individuals rediscovering the beauty of handmade, sustainable products and the joy of sharing their knowledge and skills. Soap making is just one facet of a larger movement toward more conscious living, where we embrace creativity, self-sufficiency, and the power of natural ingredients. By making your own soap, you are contributing to a greater narrative of reclaiming simplicity and authenticity in a world that often prioritizes convenience and mass production.

A Vision for the Future

I envision a future where more people embrace natural living, where local markets are filled with handmade products, and where creativity and sustainability thrive side by side. This isn't just a dream; it's a reality that's already beginning to take shape, and you are part of it. Your creations have the potential to make a difference, whether through the soaps you sell, share, or gift. You have the ability to create a ripple effect of creativity, care, and consciousness.

Inspiring Message

As you continue on this path, remember that this is just the beginning. Keep experimenting, learning, and growing. Each batch of soap you make is not merely a product; it's a reflection of your creativity, values, and journey. Continue to challenge yourself, step outside your comfort zone, and share your knowledge with others. You never know how far your creations might reach or how they may inspire someone else to start their own journey.

Quote to Inspire

"Creativity is intelligence having fun."

–Albert Einstein

Let this quote remind you that making soap—or engaging in any activity that ignites your passion—is not only a form of self-expression but also a celebration of your creativity. Stay curious, stay inspired, and never stop creating. Thank you for sharing this experience with me, and I hope your soap-making journey continues to bring you joy, fulfillment, and connection.

Wishing you all the best in your creative and natural pursuits!

www.ingramcontent.com/pod-product-compliance
Lightning Source LLC
Chambersburg PA
CBHW060230030426
42335CB00014B/1389